This book lets us hear the testimonies of the many people who have lived in the Philadelphia Association community houses. Their accounts give a fascinating insight into what it was like to have been a resident in such places. We hear of the experience of living with other people, many of whom were seriously mentally disturbed. We listen into the debates about whether medication was of value and we see how different therapists operated. The most famous, of course, was R.D. Laing who is remembered fondly by most of the residents and who comes across in these interviews as a charismatic and innovative figure, ready to engage with others. Bruce Scott sensitively frames these testimonies in the context of his wide reading of philosophy, religion and psychotherapy. The book greatly adds to our understanding of this turbulent but important era.

Dr Allan Beveridge, Consultant Psychiatrist, Queen Margaret Hospital, Dunfermline and author of *Portrait of the Psychiatrist as a Young Man. The early writings and work of R.D. Laing, 1927–1960*

Bruce Scott's book is a well-written and illuminating testimony of people's personal experiences of living within a community household. My father, R.D. Laing, was one of the co-founders of The Philadelphia Association, which set up these community houses as an alternative to conventional psychiatric wards and treatments. I highly recommend this book for anyone interested in mental health.

Karen Laing, Psychotherapist

Bruce Scott, PhD, completed his existential and phenomenologically informed training in psychoanalysis with the Philadelphia Association in London, an organisation founded by R.D. Laing and others in 1965. He is also an experimental psychologist and has conducted research into the cognitive model of depression and the cognitive effects of SSRI antidepressants. He is a member and on the Board of Governors of the College of Psychoanalysts-UK, and a member of the Philadelphia Association. He currently lives in the Scottish Borders with his wife and son. He works in private practice in the Scottish Borders and Edinburgh and continues to work as an independent writer and researcher.

Testimony of Experience

Docta Ignorantia and the Philadelphia Association Communities

Bruce Scott

PCCS Books
Ross-on-Wye

First published, 2014

PCCS BOOKS Ltd
2 Cropper Row
Alton Road
Ross-on-Wye
Herefordshire
HR9 5LA
UK
Tel +44 (0)1989 763900
www.pccs-books.co.uk

© Bruce Scott 2014

All rights reserved.

No part of this publication may be reproduced, stored in a retrieval system, transmitted or utilised in any form by any means, electronic, mechanical, photocopying or recording or otherwise, without permission in writing from the publishers.

The author has asserted his right to be identified as the author of this work in accordance with the Copyright, Designs and Patents Act 1988.

Testimony of Experience:
Docta Ignorantia **and the Philadelphia Association Communities**

A CIP catalogue record for this book is available from the British Library

ISBN 978 1 906254 64 3

Cover designed in the UK by Old Dog Graphics
Cover artwork: 'Reflections' © Bruce Scott 2013
Printed in the UK by Imprint Digital, Exeter

Contents

Preface	vii
Acknowledgements	xi
Glossary of acronyms	xii

Part One – An Incomplete Project

Chapter 1: Introducing an incomplete project — **3**
- The incomplete project — 4
- The philosophical underpinnings of the Philadelphia Association communities — 5
- The state of homelessness and the medico-scientific technicalisation of therapy — 7
- Asylum and autorhythmia — 8
- The Philadelphia Association communities and the honouring of true asylum — 11

Chapter 2: Into the paradox — **19**
- Introducing a necessary paradox — 19

Chapter 3: Method: In search of an anti-method — **22**
- The problem of scientific method — 22
- The philosophical psychology of John Macmurray: The myth of progress — 23
- The origins of Western thought: An alternative way of seeing ourselves, of living and 're-search', contra the medico-scientific psychological gaze — 28
- Parmenides, Heidegger and Levinas: The problem of psychologism, Being, and the *Other* — 29
- The problem of health — 35
- Statement for an anti-method — 41

Chapter 4: Practicalities of carrying out the research — **48**
- Data collection — 48
- Interviews — 48
- Interviewees' characteristics — 50

Part Two – Tales of *Docta Ignorantia*: Interviews with ex-residents

Chapter 5: Diana — 53
Chapter 6: Cara — 63
Chapter 7: Roland — 68
Chapter 8: Joe — 77
Chapter 9: Rob — 84
Chapter 10: Rose — 91
Chapter 11: Julia — 95
Chapter 12: Simon — 98
Chapter 13: Sally — 103
Chapter 14: Thomas — 111
Chapter 15: David — 120
Chapter 16: Peter — 127
Chapter 17: Debbie — 139
Chapter 18: Lyn — 150

Part Three – Tales of *Docta Ignorantia*: Analysis of interviews

Chapter 19: The unveiling and re-veiling of a research schema and *Docta Ignorantia*: Approaching an analysis of the interviews — 163

Introduction to *Docta Ignorantia* — 163

Analysis of interviews: Approaching *Docta Ignorantia* — 164

Chapter 20: The honesty of the perplexed and the honesty of perplexity: Analysis of interviews — 174

Part Four – Summing up a necessarily incomplete project

Chapter 21: *Meno*, Montaigne and *Docta Ignorantia* — 217

Coda — 229
Appendix — 231
References — 233
Index — 238

For

Fillan Bryn Scott

There is no hope.
There is only permanent struggle.
That is our hope.
That is a first sentence, in the language of madness.
                (David Cooper, 1978, *The Language of Madness*, p. 15)

Preface

This book is an offering of testimonies of people's experience within the context of living in a community household. Their testimony, and the comment and analysis offered in this book, hopefully go towards an understanding and *way* of 'seeing' human experience, mental distress, truth, and subjectivity, perhaps more akin to previous times and less common contexts, which is completely incongruous and incompatible with the dominant Western scientific *modus operandi*. This *way* is perilous, daunting, and possibly frustrating to a logical-positivist or scientific way of organising the world and thinking about mental distress; however, it is a great leveller and a much-needed endeavour.

As an illustration, the philosopher Levinas discussed that there is the important (and often forgotten) distinction between the *said* and the *saying* (Levinas, 1998). Some of us think we have become expert in the *said* and really believe in the transportation of signifiers being passed over from one person to another as being *the* truth, to the detriment of the almost mystical *saying* and alternative modes of truthfulness and subjectivity. This convenient but violent manoeuvre – the *conatus essendi*, the narcissistic effort and urgency towards *knowing* and *describing* being – contrary to what is being defended here, refuses other modes of subjectivity and truthfulness. This is especially pertinent in the realm of mental distress, for where there are people in power, and people who want power, there cannot be anything other than the proliferation of the *conatus essendi*, misery and misunderstanding due to the authoritarian foreclosure of alternative modes of subjectivity and truthfulness. Considering this power differential, it is no wonder some people in distress get lost, slowly wither, or leave the 'system', opt out, and try to make their own way or find others (or not) with whom to traverse life's journey. Some are lucky enough to come to the realisation that there is more to life or something richer than just the *said* as a way to truthfulness, authenticity, or subjecthood.

The recent publication of the new and 'improved' *Diagnostic and Statistical Manual of Mental Disorders* (*DSM-5*, American Psychiatric Association, 2013) is a case in point, of misunderstanding and authoritarian foreclosure of alternative ways of conceptualising mental distress and human experience. This is a serious matter: the violence done to the diversity of experience under the guise of the rhetoric of the *DSM*, purely by the words that are written in it, read by people, and transported from one who is supposed to know to another in the guise of helping, is truly astounding. Moreover, when the layman (or any man or woman) has only a *DSM*-esque taxonomical discourse to light their way, it is no wonder that many get shipwrecked; however, despite what some people say, there are other paths.

This book attempts to show some people who have made their own way (sometimes with the help of others) and are making their way on routes and paths that are becoming less and less available to others as a result of the state's and related institutions' definitions and management of mental distress. Slowly and surely the discourse of the capitalist, the bureaucrat, the call to 'accountability', certainty, predictability, are all shoring up the *surplus* that such divergent pathmakers stir up and which such discourses cannot really, ever truly account for.

This book, and it is of paramount importance for me to express this, is not a presentation in the sense of a 'Here is how you do it'. Perhaps Wittgenstein provides a good example of my sentiments. In the *Tractatus Logico-Philosophicus* he writes:

> 6.52: We feel that even when all possible scientific questions have been answered, the problems of life remain completely untouched. Of course there are then no questions left, and this itself is the answer.
>
> 6.521: The solution of the problem of life is seen in the vanishing of the problem. (Is this not the reason why those who have found after a long period of doubt that the sense of life became clear to them have been unable to say what constituted that sense?)
>
> 6.522: There are things that cannot be put into words. They make themselves manifest. They are what is mystical.
>
> (Wittgenstein, 1961, p. 73)

Indeed, taking this seriously, perhaps Wittgenstein's wisdom reflects the importance of the title of this book; that testimony and *Docta Ignorantia*[1] (*learned* ignorance or wise unknowing) are beyond ideals of representation; they are a call to the ethical, to justice, to freedom. The dominant Western psycho-scientific research and philosophical outlooks proceed on the basis of the desire for the understanding of beings or entities; of intelligibility. But as Levinas argues, such drive for intelligibility is questionable:

> Consequently truth is a progression, and is exposed in several moments, remaining problematical in each. Yet the question about the question is more radical still. Why does research take form as a question? How is it that the 'what', already steeped in being so as to open it up the more, becomes a demand and a prayer, a special language inserting into 'communication' of the given an appeal for help, for aid addressed to another?
>
> (Levinas, 1998, p. 24)

So the question is: why does there have to be this incessant call for the intelligible, for the question mark put in the service of research, in the context of mental distress? Of course I am not demeaning mental distress or romanticising misery; I am championing mental distress as a facet of life that should not be swept under the carpet or got rid of, as mental distress is an important guiding facet of living. The vicissitudes of life are multifarious and infinitely changeable. My point is that all is life; happiness, suffering and everything in between; all is needed, it is all part of (what should be expected of) experience. Language or discourse is not a neutral, benign, or always helpful aid; we are all beings suffused with the cultural signifiers of our time. We have to question the question before we end up tumbling down a rabbit hole where there might be no end to the riddles we encounter.

One can read this book throughout as a whole, or one could read the individual chapters as standalone pieces. Readers without specialist philosophical knowledge can omit Chapters 2, 3, or 19 if they wish. By reading the interview chapters alone (Chapters 5–18) along with the analysis in Chapter 20, one can gain a more than adequate insight into the experiences I wish to convey. It is the *testimony* that is contained within this book which I hope the reader will be open to; not as a grasping after fact, but as letting it change and work on them. The testimony, from my own hand (and from those that have inspired me), and especially from the people I interviewed who have lived in the Philadelphia Association communities, will hopefully open up a poetic dwelling space where the constraints of certainty are loosened and the realm of *Docta Ignorantia* is honoured. Life is not a technique, and life is not here to be 'known'; young children are more aware of this than adults I believe; this cannot be taught in a lecture or PowerPoint presentation, however clever we think we are. I think there has to be more room in life for poetising, even in the realm of mental distress and psychotherapeutic work. If such poetising is cultured out, as it seems to be today, we will be witnesses to the refusal of testimony in its true sense; to be witness to the vicissitudes of life, *Docta Ignorantia* or wise unknowing. Testimony is not towards a 'truth' but rather towards a truthfulness of living life that can never be fully spoken; this is the wonderfulness of poetry and of life.

Bruce Scott
Jedburgh
May 2013

Endnote

1. *Docta Ignorantia* was a concept used by Nicolaus Cusanus, a fifteenth-century theologian and philosopher (Cusanus, 2007). *Docta Ignorantia* originated in the ideas of Parmenides and Plato and today traces of it remain in the likes of Kierkegaard, Wittgenstein, Derrida, and the psychoanalyst Jacques Lacan. Cusanus demonstrated how 'finite' thought is limited and betrays our fundamental capacities of (or *for*) not-knowing and the infinitude of *Being* that constantly get sidelined when we place finitude upon the world via our scientistic posturing. Cusanus demonstrated our fundamental wrong-turning of relying upon human intellect by showing through the examples of comparing and contrasting finite and infinite lines, circles and triangles, how our limited human conceptualisation and cogitation can only *reveal* to a certain point.

Acknowledgements

There are too many people to thank.

Thank you to: Paul Gordon and the Philadelphia Association for the encouragement of this study and James Low, John Heaton, Noel Cobb, and Julia Evans for being great 'teachers', each in their own different ways. The current house therapists from the Philadelphia Association, Paul Gordon, Ian Macmillan, Jake Osborne and Hilary Cooper, for the wisdom and common sense they have shown to me in their respective and varied ways, in relation to my contact with them and the PA communities; also thank you for keeping the communities going. Thank you to Theodor Itten who encouraged me to write. I also owe a great deal of gratitude to Francis Gillett for his wisdom and insight into the PA communities. Thank you to Janet Haney for introducing me and opening my eyes to the world of regulation in action and its effects on the 'talking therapies'. Thank you to my friends, colleagues and comrades in the Philadelphia Association, the Alliance for Psychotherapy and Counselling, the Psychoanalytic Consortium, Lacanian Works, and the College of Psychoanalysts–UK, for their passion, wisdom, and their dedication to the protection of the work that we do. I must thank Bruno de Florence, Jo Rostron, and Julia Evans of the Earls Court Lacanian Cartel for letting me discuss many of the ideas that are within this book and being able to learn so much from their valuable wisdom and feedback. Without the testimony of the interviewees there would be no book; I thank them from the bottom of my heart for baring their souls and sharing their time with me – at last the ex-residents have their testimony. Thank you all at PCCS Books for all the work of producing this book and having faith in its content: especially Heather Allen, Director of PCCS Books; Sandy Green, copy-editor; Sam Taylor, typesetting; and Jonathan Hopkins, proofreader. Nothing I do or write about is done in a vacuum; thank you to my loving and supportive friends and family and my wonderful Clare and Fillan. I am also grateful to Bosch for the memories and guidance, and Cooper et al. for the language of madness.

Glossary of acronyms

CBT: cognitive behavioural therapy

CHRE: Council for Healthcare Regulatory Excellence (now PSA)

DSM: Diagnostic and Statistical Manual of Mental Disorders

HCPC: the HPC changed its name in 2012 to the Health and Care Professions Council

HPC: Health Professions Council (now HCPC)

IAPT: Improving Access to Psychological Therapies

NICE: National Institute for Health and Care Excellence

PA: Philadelphia Association

PSA: CHRE was renamed the Professional Standards Authority (for Health and Social Care) in November 2012

Part 1

An incomplete project

Chapter One

Introducing an incomplete project[1]

Fortune's demand brought to me the opportunity of researching the experience of people who have lived in Philadelphia Association community houses. Little has been written about the topic of the experience of living in a PA community household before, especially in the way I set out to do it: to interview ex-residents and explore the narratives of what they thought about their experiences. In many ways, for many people the nature of the houses and what they 'do' is clouded in mystery, secrecy, or unknowing. This may or may not be a bad thing; indeed to proceed on groundlessness and to end on groundlessness may be the only and right way to undertake such a project as this. The package, the theory and the formula for 'curing' mental distress causes so much trouble for people. Because of this, it is surprising there is such a demand for it. The demand has been argued to be the problem; it is like the Zen idea of washing blood with blood, which relates the foolish idea of trying to wash away bad thoughts with more thoughts, which only leads back to square one – covered in blood or more bad thoughts. So fortune's demand put me in a tricky position: I may be damned if I do and damned if I don't; to provide or not provide a theory from the results of this research project. But I always had a nagging doubt that there may be another way or another path around this problem. This was not clear to begin with. Indeed, I had many months of struggle, sadness, writer's block, confusion, misery, boredom, and joy at times when dealing with the project. It was then that it hit me; in many ways I had embodied the experience of those who had actually lived in a PA house, perhaps to lesser degree, but nevertheless the struggle of living in a PA community house. I too, like many ex-residents of PA communities, was looking for an 'answer' or 'meaning' that ended up being quite elusive and destructive at times. It took me a while to realise I had to find my own path in the project, but that the struggle was a necessary part of the deal. I just had to learn and wait and be patient. One cannot learn patience from books or theories and one certainly cannot write about it as a formula to be mechanically applied or used like a tool. That is just like washing blood off with more blood. As Meister Eckhart said in relation to the spiritual path, which is also applicable to the human condition:

> The spiritual path doesn't require us to get anything. It's a process of opening to new dimensions of who we already are. It's a process of awakening to our own truth. It's a process of allowing ourselves to be authentic.
>
> (Eckhart, in Evans, 1924, p. 38)

Eckhart's wisdom is a starting point to meditate upon, and a possible end point, but in actuality there is no ending; such a path or praxis is never ending. The teleology of praxis, as Aristotle (see Dunne, 1993) beautifully put it, has no end-point goal, such as when one attempts to produce a result on finishing a task; the act of praxis is steadfast in the action of doing the action for its own sake, not for a point in the future or future product. That is why neatly packaged theories about how to cure mental distress fall into error – teleological processes (seeking a product), end-point goals and formulas provide an illusion of an end point. As Plato (in Cooper, 1997) said, we cannot ever grasp 'The One'; it is without parts, out of time, it is not one, not many, nor of shape, colour, or weight. For many of us, our Western scientific minds baulk at such a statement. However, if we are mindful enough of what Plato had to say on the matter, it just might bear fruit or at least open up a different kind of 'path', as opposed to the Western scientific dogmatic bias to the logos of empiricism. Heidegger (1977) argued that this aspect of 'Being', in our present technological age, had been forgotten and neglected. It was these issues (as well as much more) that brought people together in London back in the mid-1960s to form the Philadelphia Association and set up community households. Their concern is just as relevant today as it was then (perhaps now even more relevant and urgent). This is why I took up fortune's demand of taking on an incomplete project.

The incomplete project

Beginning the project of finding out what the Philadelphia Association community houses are all about was very tricky. For a start, as is the nature of the PA, keeping records of residents was not a major priority; there were (and rightly so) much more important things to attend to. But as the PA has veered into the twenty-first century, 45 years after its creation, events are occurring in our society and culture at large that concern issues pertaining not just to mental distress, but also to human freedom, and which have necessitated the voices of those who found asylum in the PA and its communities to be heard.

The Philadelphia Association was set up by R.D. Laing and others in 1965 as a response to the treatment of people in the psychiatric system and to reductionism regarding the ideas about mental illness that prevailed in the 1960s. Put simply, Laing and others fought for the space of therapy, a place for asylum, and for therapists and patients to be protected, not violated, and for human rights to be defended. This resulted in the creation of the famous Kingsley Hall community in East London, the very first 'official' PA community household. Forty-five years later, we live in a curious world where the PA's championing of psychotherapy, community and asylum over psychiatric treatment seems, on the surface, to have had some impact. Today we have the government-run Improving Access to Psychological Therapies (IAPT), the National Institute for Health and Care Excellence (NICE), cognitive behavioural therapy (CBT), Care in the Community, the Supporting People Programme, the Health and Care Professions Council (HCPC)[2] and the Professional Standards Authority (PSA),[3] the latter two both being keen to see the regulation and professionalism of all the psychotherapies and all kinds of 'psychotherapeutic endeavours'. Sounds great does it not?

However, in our current times of the early twenty-first century, I believe something seems to have gone awry in the world. The hope of the 1960s seems to have been developed into a narcissistic demand (from some quarters)[4] that wants all mental distress, patients (or 'service users'[5]) and therapists of all modalities to be objectified, regulated, controlled, and predictable. The message espoused by the PA in the 1960s was that 'authentic being' (e.g., Heidegger, 2001) is never a solidified, concrete, objective reality, but a living, breathing and forever-evolving way of living; a *praxis* whose teleology is contra a teleology inherent in *poiesis*. In other words the art of therapy is beyond a process/product orientation, and is instead a practice where the activity itself is of value and for the sake of it. Today's demand for a product and outcome totalisation/conceptualisation in dealing with mental distress, patients and therapists represents Levinas's (2007) worst nightmare.

The philosophical underpinnings of the Philadelphia Association communities

The radical thought that underpinned the conception of the houses I believe has its roots in the ideas of certain philosophers[6] (see Mullan, 1995). One such philosopher was Friedrich Nietzsche. His ideas on suffering and those who help are and were very much present in the

PA houses and could be regarded as being a critique of modern day psychiatry and mental health care. Nietzsche sums this up very well in *The Gay Science* in Book Four, section 338: 'The will to suffer and those who feel pity'. This passage explains the naïvety of trying to do something to somebody to get them out of his or her hell. He asks:

> Is it good for you yourselves to be above all full of pity? And is it good for those who suffer?
>
> (Nietzsche, 1974, p. 269)

He goes on to describe the helper who tries to help the person in distress:

> When people try to benefit someone in distress, the intellectual frivolity with which those moved by pity assume the role is for the most part outrageous; one simply knows nothing of the whole inner sequence and intricacies that are distress for me or you ... they wish to help and have no thought of the personal necessity of distress, although terrors, deprivations, impoverishments, midnights, adventures, risks, and blunders are as necessary for you as are their opposites. It never occurs to them that, to put it mystically, the path to one's own heaven always leads through the voluptuousness of one's own hell.
>
> (Nietzsche, 1974, p. 269)

Nietzsche blames this idea on the religion of comfortableness and the rush to extinguish someone's pain:

> ... if you refuse to let your own suffering lie upon you for even an hour and if you constantly try to prevent and forestall all possible distress ... it is clear that besides the religion of pity you also harbour another religion in your heart ... the religion of comfortableness. ... How little you know of human happiness, you comfortable and benevolent people, for happiness and unhappiness are sisters and even twins that either grow up together or, as in your case, remain small together.
>
> (Nietzsche, 1974, pp. 269–270)

The point I am trying to labour through the philosophy of Nietzsche is that Laing and his colleagues within the Philadelphia Association saw the value in not arresting someone's distress. Indeed, it was regarded as naïve to suppress distress because if one did pursue this course of action, psychological growth or development would be impeded as a result. Further, the idea of the helper, jumping in and trying to do things to stop the pain, is tantamount to violence (Buber, 1970; Levinas, 1998, 2007). This is because, in essence, owing to the automatic instinct to stop anything negative, it does not let be said what is meant to be said, does not let something open that has to be opened up and dwelt upon for the individual concerned. Laing (1967) was correct in that psychiatry was silencing people's distress, not letting them be heard, and treating people like objects as a result of a totalising psychiatric discourse and power which overruled the life, feelings, and thoughts of those who were in distress. In other words, Laing felt that a place like a PA house would allow people to go through whatever they probably should go through and that they would not be silenced and coerced by well-meaning people who think that all mental pain is bad just because they have the technology and ability to get rid of it through various neurochemical anaesthetics (i.e., drugs).

However, the lay public and many people within psychotherapy and psychiatric societies are completely aghast at the suggestion of letting someone go into a household where no *treatment* will be given or done to people – they just *can't get it*. It appears therefore that we still do live by the religion of comfortableness where mental pain is immediately regarded as negative and it is our right to be rid of such things.

The state of homelessness and the medico-scientific technicalisation of therapy

The problem, I feel, and which Laing and colleagues were keenly aware of, is that many of us in the advanced capitalist West are to a great extent cut off, alienated, numb, and essentially living in a state of homelessness. This is caused to a large degree by the way we live, the way we see the world and think what it has to offer, and the way we treat ourselves and others. Another way of conceptualising this state of affairs is that the majority of institutions and government bodies in the so-called service of those in mental distress operate within either the position of Lacan's discourse of the university and/or aspects attributed to (depending on the hierarchical, social or political context) the discourse of the hysteric and/or master. This closes down the idea of a free subject, and allowing an individual's own path to develop (Lacan, 2007). This is the value of the PA houses and what they offered and offer for all the 'homeless' people who have come to the houses: a place to become less cut off and more connected.

By 'homeless' I am referring to ideas of dwelling and homelessness beautifully described by Robin Cooper in a chapter called 'Dwelling and the Therapeutic Community' from the book *Thresholds between Philosophy and Psychoanalysis* (Cooper et al., 1994). Cooper describes the way in which individuals who arrive at the PA community houses are unsure in their being, and feel they have little freedom to move and move around: in other words, not knowing one's way and not feeling at home in and around the world; in essence, not having a safe sense of the world which could be called being at home with oneself. However, a building with *therapy being done in it to people* does not instil in the resident a sense of home (e.g., the Richmond Fellowship or a psychiatric ward, see Itten, 1977). In other words, the idea of a therapeutic programme where social skills, well-being, positive-thought reprogramming, relaxation techniques, budgeting, house management and so on are taught and carried out by rote – to produce rehabilitated individuals to return to the *community* to live alone in their self-contained sterile existences – does not and cannot instil a sense of being at home with oneself.

Heidegger (2001) explains very well why this is the case. He asserts that any therapeutic endeavour cannot be formalised as such to instil a sense of home in an individual. If one believes that psychotherapy can only be done if one objectifies the human being (as modern psychiatry and the mental health care system do), then what is decisive is the psychotherapy and not the existence of the human being. If this is so, the practice of psychotherapy would resemble a procedure concerned only with the handling of an object, and thus something purely technical. The outcome of such psychotherapy cannot result in a healthier human being. In psychotherapy conducted in this way, the best result can only be a more polished object. I am reminded at this point of something written by David Cooper (1978), a past member of the PA, now deceased: he asserted that norms impose needs, they do not recognise them. So if we are treated like objects, then these treatments will impose the needs of the treatment, to the detriment of any recognition of our own needs.

Asylum and autorhythmia

This leads me to the issues of autorhythmia (self-regulation) and asylum, historically very much key elements of the PA houses, and a direct negation of an objectifying way of treating someone in mental distress. Leon Redler (2000) describes that Kingsley Hall, the first PA house, was founded on the principle of asylum. Redler asks us to consider what we would like to happen to us or how we would like to be treated if we ended up 'schizophrenic'. He explains that the Kingsley Hall experiment and the PA were not emphasising the 'treatment of schizophrenia', but the way we treat each other. The ethos was that the way we treat each other is very important. This is of paramount importance whether or not there is a biochemical, physiological, or genetic irregularity correlated with the development of schizophrenia. If there are such correlates, the way in which we treat each other probably has much to do with development of the schizophrenia. Therefore, treatment should not be based on the premise of objectification, as that is far too one-sided and overly technical, as Heidegger (2001) argued. The asylum provided by a PA house would be one in which one would not be treated like an object; the environment would be one of *being with* rather than *doing to*, a place where one could entrust one's being into the care of others.

So how was/is this kind of place meant to help by not doing? Robin Cooper (in Cooper et al., 1994) suggested the term *autorhythmia* to describe finding one's way or how to be at home in one's own being. This would involve nothing out of the ordinary. A person may find their own rhythm at their own pace and in their own time. They may seek outside therapy if they wish, they may get a job, they may sleep, or they may eat fish and chips when they want. This is the essence of autorhythmia. This way or path is the distinct reversal of perhaps the strict requirements (time, space, relationships, work, etc.) of the life that was led by the person which contributed to a state of breakdown in the first place. Thus when the old life structure breaks down, as PA therapist Joe Friedman argues in his chapter called '*Therapeia*, Play and the Therapeutic Household' (in Cooper et al., 1994), it is helpful to be free of the structural constraints that got the person into a knot originally, to bring a person back into a state of play, a less egoic way of being, with the awareness that we are all in the same boiling pot together; *so we have to get on together as we are not really different or separated*; we as a species all suffer from the same struggles of everyday life, how to live a good life, and the human condition. To recognise this is to recognise that we all have to make a concerted and collective effort to get out of the cut-off, alienated state that Laing believed us to be in. A technical approach to psychotherapy, at the very least, destroys possibilities of getting out of our cut-off or alienated state.

In the following quote, R.D. Laing (1977) expresses what the PA houses were all about and clearly explains the non-psycho-technical environment of the houses:

> Suppose you freak out, have a nervous breakdown, come to the end of your tether, go to pieces, can no longer cope. It can happen to anyone. Where would you go? To whom would you turn?
>
> Suppose you do not want to be jolted out of it, but believe that this is something you want to go through. Who will allow you to go through it? Where will you be allowed to plumb the depths of agony, despair, bewilderment, confusion, perplexity, until a new beginning dawns? No one is asking you to, if you don't want to. But just supposing you feel you have to? ...

> Suppose one is looking for a refuge from all the advice and treatment proposed or imposed by our well-intentioned parents, teachers, doctors, rulers and revolutionaries, who all think they know best for us.
>
> Then one wants an asylum, a safe place, a sanctuary, a shelter. There, one can have, if one wants, a pleasant room of one's own, while other people see to it that there is food, warmth, and shelter, and try to hold the balance between care, concern, attention, and letting be ...
>
> They (the houses) have all been melting pots, crucibles in which many, if not all, of our initial assumptions about normal–abnormal, conformist–deviant, sane–crazy experience and behaviour have been dissolved ...
>
> With no staff, 'patients', or institutional procedures, behaviour is feasible which is intolerable in most other places. People get up or stay in bed as they wish, eat what they want, stay alone or be with others and generally make their own rules.
>
> These are places where people can be together and let each other be.
> (Laing, 1977, excerpt from Philadelphia Association leaflet)

A view taken by a current member of the PA and friend of the late R.D. Laing, Theodor Itten (1977), describes the difficulty of defining what the PA houses and the PA are all about:

> What is the PA? It is an association of people. Not directly an institution, nor an organisation, at least not in the way this term is generally understood in our society. Organising is a making sense of something that is already happening. And in this sense, the PA and all the people currently involved in it, in all their ways, are an organisation. What is the PA on about? R.D. Laing ... has said that we can't entirely say what we are all on about. We are involved in something to do with suffering to let it happen and ways and means to make it happen, so that one experiences it, in its bottom, and is able to go through it and walk one's path, which no-one else will ever walk for oneself.
> (Itten, 1977, p. 1)

Itten goes on to describe the views of Medard Boss:

> His [Boss's] work, of which I can only present a small glimpse, is also an example of one of the European thinkers which had some influence on Laing. Boss brings together in his writings an

all-embracing and fundamental outline of what the pre-scientific foundation of any study of human phenomena is; that is, if one really wants to really and meaningfully support one's fellow human beings, and heal them from the bottom upwards, one must by oneself first have gained clarity about what actually the human being in his/her true essence is, and how and what she/he is. Otherwise one remains forever a quack doctor and wanders helplessly in the dark with all attempts to cure.

(Itten, 1977, pp. 3–4)

Boss said at our meeting that he is not claiming that his way is the only way, but for him, with experience of psychoanalytical and analytical psychological practice and thought, this is the most human and liberating understanding of meaningful living. He [Boss] pointed out, in respect to the PA's work, that it is a worthwhile venture and a long way ahead of other treatment centres.

(Itten, 1977, p. 4)

The Philadelphia Association communities and the honouring of true asylum[7]

The project of writing about the PA communities is also very difficult for another reason – the PA communities are unique in that similar 'therapeutic communities' work from different protocols, assumptions, models, and beliefs of how and why one should help those in mental distress.

In the PA communities, as in other communities, people share space and time; this is a given when people come together and live together, whether they like sharing the space and time together or even *want* to share it. Holding this together are the actual walls of the house. As Itten (1977) describes, community is where true community and sharing are sporadic and not something constant. It is, he argues, the moments in such places where 'doing one's own thing' is seen as the only hope for people to be able to express their individuality in a mass society like ours. This experience of individuality is not egotism. Rather as Ross Speck argues:

The almost total acceptance of one another's differences and their right to do their own thing is probably the outstanding component [of therapeutic communities].

(Speck, 1974, p. 74)

And these moments of 'finding oneself', although perhaps rare or not-so-rare (varying from individual to individual and community to community), show the nature of community and how its foundation rests upon the dialectic of stability and instability. It is a living system in flux; the community might die and fade away if ideals of a 'constant' are put into place, if ideological borders are fixed, or so-called emancipatory projects with fixed representations are dictated (Balibar, 1999; Derrida, 1997).

Looking at Foucault's idea of an asylum might help our way forward here. Foucault unpicks the meaning of the word 'asylum'; that it is an unassailable sanctuary, refuge and retreat for the persecuted. It aids the retreat and concrete experience of madness, in its ideal setting. However, as any cursory glance at the history of psychiatric asylums shows, this meaning of asylum was hardly implemented (Foucault, 2001, 2008).

As a result of his research in this area, Itten (1977) believes that the Philadelphia Association communities come closest to the ideal of asylum. However, before we venture as to why this is so, let us first explore the nature of asylum in hospital settings as described by Foucault (2001, 2008), and Itten's (1977) research of another community, the Richmond Fellowship.

Foucault (2008) outlines in his lectures at the Collège de France (1973–1974) how the strange function of the nineteenth-century psychiatric hospital was established as a site for diagnosis and classification. This still exists today and in other 'communities' associated with mental distress (e.g., Rethink).[8] The different species of disease and disorder are laid out around the hospital (e.g., eating disorders unit, personality disorder, schizophrenic/acute psychosis wards). This creates an enclosed space for confrontation, the site of a duel, an institutional field where victory and submission are at stake. Foucault contends that this kind of asylum sets up the doctors (or psychiatrists, psychiatric nurses, auxiliary staff, albeit hierarchically) as seers of the truth of the illness through the knowledge they have of it and the fact they can produce the illness in its truth and subjugate it in reality through the power the doctor's will exerts over the patient. The techniques or procedures of the asylum or psychiatric system such as isolation (isolation rooms for acute psychosis), public (ward rounds) and private (meetings with a psychiatrist) cross-examination, treatment-punishments (very strong sedatives for behaviour that is unwanted, or disobedience of rules), discipline (banning hospital leave) and rewards (hospital leave for good behaviour), which bind a patient to the psychiatrist, are very prevalent today in psychiatric hospitals.[9] As Foucault points out, the function of this structure is to make the medical figurehead (i.e., the psychiatrist) the 'master of madness'; the person who makes it appear in its truth,[10] and the person who dominates it, pacifies it, and cures it after having created it. This situation would be laudable if it were the only 'truth' that cures and guides those in a state of madness and distress, but clearly this is not the only truth. To digress from Foucault for a minute, I would like to describe a (common) story of a survivor of the mental health system where this situation is shown clearly.

A young woman went to university and during her studies experienced a very acrimonious break-up from her boyfriend. Of course grief and depression set in over a period of a few weeks, and a visit to her GP did not confirm 'ordinary grief' but abnormal serotonin levels thus needing pills to correct this. Submitting to the 'superior' knowledge of the GP, the woman took the pills for a while, eventually becoming addicted to them. It took some time for her to wean herself off the pills. However, later this woman found a sympathetic therapist who bore no real 'truth' other than he was willing to be a witness to the woman and her grief. The woman's suicidal impulses were listened to, no outside intervention (interference) was called, there was no attempt to stop her pain, and no assertions to cure were posited: a crazy and irresponsible situation some may argue. After about one year into analysis three times a week, it suddenly dawned on this woman that there was no cure. Yes, no cure. Some might think this a ludicrous conclusion. However, looked at from a different standpoint (or truth) what was there to be cured? The discourse of psychiatric truth that had held this woman in its grip (e.g., happiness resembles an obtainable object; the self should be malleable like an object; low moods are negative and should be eradicated by enhancing serotonin levels/regulation) had loosened. She no longer believed in this neuro-cognitive dogma. This was, ironically, her cure. To believe that there was no cure, contrary to the standpoint of a psychiatric definition of truth of what depression is, was in fact the cure. She had found her own truth. To find one's own truth in the asylum is very difficult when you have a master of madness telling you what the truth is.

David Cooper (1978) – a founding member of the Philadelphia Association – argued that the heart of this problem of defining truth in regards to 'mental health' is nothing other than violence; a violence on the power of the dialectic of truth. For in such a context (i.e., the psychiatric system), where is the opportunity for a patient to create his or her own truth? In other words, would a psychiatrist accept the reliability of a patient's account that there is no cure for depression, thus telling the psychiatrist that his or her knowledge or theories of depression are meaningless and false for them (i.e., for the patient)? If the psychiatrist retorted that some people benefited from the medico-scientific intervention in depression for example, that is fine for those people who had benefited, but for someone who does not subscribe to this notion, then it is not applicable and thus very unhelpful. This is the crux of the problem when it comes to the assertions of the masters of madness; they assert that their truth is the only valid and reliable truth.

Returning to Foucault (2001, 2008), the birth of the modern psychiatric hospital served as a function of truth about the nature of madness. Indeed perhaps the modern psychiatric system has moved on from punishing people for their madness, but it has moved into the realm of organising madness and people with mental distress. This change is a passage from a world of censure (e.g., locked up in a madhouse never to be seen again), to a world of judgement. In a modern-day psychiatric hospital, the work done by its patients becomes deprived of any productive value.[11] The hospital is then merely a place where a moral rule of society is carried out (e.g., what depression is and how it should be treated). It thus places a limitation on liberty (to find one's own truth) and a submission to order (e.g., how to order your experience).

This philosophy flourishes in many therapeutic communities today. For example, as Itten (1977) describes, in the Richmond Fellowship, if one could get a job and hold it down for an adequate period of time, one was considered by staff as half-cured. Being able to work was glorified and people were pushed into jobs, however meaningless they were. In the PA houses, as current PA house therapist Paul Gordon (2010) describes, residents in the past and present were/are not pushed into jobs for the sake of getting a job. A resident may be encouraged to take up a job if that is what the resident wishes, but their motivations for getting the job may be questioned in the house meetings or by their personal therapist. As many psychotherapists and psychoanalysts might argue, getting a job may imply many different things other than wanting to make money. People take jobs for all kinds of reasons: power, egocentric concerns, martyrdom, workaholism, to escape facing their problems, to fulfil parental demands, and so on. I am not arguing that work per se is bad, but work needs to be questioned in regard to all its complex facets; why one is doing it, what one's motivations are, what the ethics of the actual work are, why one must do such and such a kind of work or even work at all, etc. These questions go way beyond the purely financial necessity of work.

Taking into account the structural analysis of therapeutic communities compared to the Philadelphia Association, Itten (1977) describes how 'control' in non-PA communities rests with the staff. Staff control affects the control of the environment, freedom of movement, authority and decision making, control over personal time and self-expression, communication and behaviour, self-experience and experience of others. Foucault (2001, 2008) concurs with this scenario, describing how, within an 'institutional' environment like a psychiatric hospital ward or care in the community, something is born which is no longer repression (for indeed mental illness is recognised), but authority.[12] Mental illness therefore becomes a minority status and those deemed 'mentally ill' do not have the right of autonomy (although lip service is paid to 'service-user autonomy'). Goffman (1974), concurring with this idea, argues that institutions can disrupt or defile self-selected expressive behaviour which is the symbol of self-determination. In other words, inmates, residents or 'service users', as well as employees, are made to display a giving-up of their will.

Institutions today, such as psychiatric wards in hospitals or supported housing/care in the community, are environments not of healing but of domination, totalisation, and infantilism. Mental illness, or those who are purported to suffer from one of the *Diagnostic and Statistical Manual*'s mental disorders (APA, 2013), is guided in an authoritarian way, leading to a so-called ethical uniformity, a preordained and prearranged version of normality which a person will have to fit into to be judged 'well' or 'mentally healthy'.

Maxwell Jones (in Rapoport, 2001), who was a pioneer of the development of communities for those in mental distress and also an advisor to the Philadelphia Association in its early days, argued that it is very clear that the social environment of psychiatric patients, whether in hospital or in the outside community, can have a profound effect on their re-adjustment and eventual recovery. But as Itten (1977) points out, recovery has connotations of replacing one thing with another, hiding something, protection and pretence. Many commentators on the social injustices meted out to those classified as mentally ill (i.e., Foucault, 2001, 2008; Deleuze & Guattari, 2004) agree that although such tactics of recovery may get one out of a mental institution, they are tactics that insidiously take away our freedom. As Deleuze and Guattari (2004) eloquently argue, conforming to concepts and models of mental illness and normality, whether in a psychiatric hospital, a therapeutic community, or in so-called 'normal or sane' community care surroundings, is a dangerous action and not what should be done in the pursuit of living a good life, but more importantly, a free life.

This point shows how this incomplete project of trying to write about the Philadelphia Association communities and those who have lived in them becomes very problematic. We have come across the danger of dangers – the totalising framework which denies the paradox – the paradox being the difficulty in prescribing a theory of treatment for mental distress, as the technological application of such a theory can be bound up with power and the limitation of freedom. This is why saying anything about people's experiences in a PA community is a questionable endeavour, and perhaps also why so little has been written about the PA communities. There is inherent is this project an impossibility of saying anything which one will be able to apply in the manner of a rigid formula. If one did do such a thing, a foreclosure, a cutting-off of the possibilities of subjectivity on the part of readers, researchers and recipients of such a theory would be the result. This is why even a qualitative approach (as a comforting humanistic retreat from a quantitative approach – people as people rather than statistics), whereby categories of meaning are ascertained from people's narratives and harvested and refined for tidy analysis and speculation, is fraught with difficulty and can lead to further research studies which also fall short. But what is the alternative? Perhaps we have to take Feyerabend's (1975) lead and proceed counter-inductively. Kierkegaard (1975) believed that letting oneself be taken over with the paradox actually leads to freedom, whereas to fight the paradox leads to repetition and imprisonment in a methodological fixation which does not lead to a human flourishing. I explore this further in the next section.

Endnotes

1. This title is based on the title of Chris Oakley's opening chapter in the Philadelphia Association-produced book *Thresholds between Philosophy and Psychoanalysis* (Cooper et al., 1994).
2. The Health and Care Professions Council (HCPC) was formerly known as the Health Professions Council (HPC) before 1 August 2012.
3. The Professional Standards Authority was known as the Council for Healthcare Regulatory Excellence (CHRE) before 30 November 2012.
4. The recent demands from the Health and Care Professions Council (HCPC) and Professional Standards Authority are that all 'talking therapies' and related 'psychotherapeutic endeavours should be regulated; neatly packaged and formulated within medico-scientific guidelines. These demands could be understood from the Lacanian framework, indicating the faltering symbolic discourse associated with the discourse of the hysteric, master, or university. It is a matter of debate which discourse is dominant, or the order or process of usurpation of one discourse for another. Suffice to say however, the demand for certainty that drives these institutions' projects is wholly unsuitable for the purposes of dealing with mental distress. See Lacan (2007).
5. I detest the term 'service users' as it is commonly used in the psychiatric and mental health industry. It perhaps is indicative of how the vast majority of mental health institutions and policy makers that cater for those in mental distress see human interaction: of somebody getting something

from another, of using them. However, when it boils down to the crux of the matter, therapists, psychologists, psychiatrists, support workers, and patients are being used by a discourse that guides them and consequently robs one of truly meeting another person.

6. Other philosophers who were studied included Søren Kierkegaard, Jean-Paul Sartre, Martin Heidegger, and Michel de Montaigne, to name a few that the Philadelphia Association co-founders were inspired by.

7. The kind of asylum I am referring to is not the culturally misled idea of a lunatic asylum and all the horrors that entails. I am referring to (as do the PA) to the Latin *asylum* 'sanctuary', from Greek *asylon* 'refuge', related to the ideas of being inviolable, safe from violence, especially of persons seeking protection, from right of seizure. So literally 'an inviolable place'.

8. Rethink is an organisation that follows the dogma of 'biological mental illness' and the associated *Diagnostic and Statistical Manual of Mental Disorders (DSM)*. Fact sheets obtained from their website instruct viewers on the nature of the myriad of mental illnesses as though the information they provide is cast in stone and there is no other way or method of approaching the topic (see www.rethink.org) Such organisations, like many others (e.g., NHS, NICE, HCPC), view mental illness in this way, whilst ignoring evidence which challenges such a dogmatic approach. For example, Moncrieff (2003) and Healy (2003) have both provided strong critiques of the biological model.

9. This is based upon the author's experience of working in several psychiatric hospitals.

10. The truth in this sense is one version of the truth. Psychiatric truth is a shaky truth, with methodological difficulties and difficulties of verification plaguing the profession and discipline. Two examples are the serotonin hypothesis of depression and the dopamine hypothesis of schizophrenia; both are refutable yet act as a mainstay of psychiatric practice both in and out of the institution of the hospital (see Healy, 2003, and Moncrieff, 2003).

11. Perhaps the staff's work is also devoid of any *productive* (or I would prefer to say, human) value. This lack of human value is present in many psychiatric hospital wards and in the supported housing units that arose from the shambolic and ideologically lame UK government's initiative for care in the community (where residents share a house but do not communicate

with each other and where there is no trust, for example, residents having separate locked cupboards for food in their shared houses). For the most part, the panoptic bureaucratic structure of 'care in the community' supported housing/outreach projects consists of staff endlessly filling in forms, completing care plans, and producing risk assessments; this is where the bulk of producing takes place. If one chooses to call this a *productive* or a humane working system for trying to help people in mental distress, then it is no wonder that relating to another human being on each other's terms may seem to the advocates of the psycho-bureaucracy as pointless and irresponsible, especially in light of their thoughtless and ill-informed dogma centred on 'duty of care'. Is it not the responsibility of staff to question what their duty actually is and what it means to care about themselves, their working environment, and also how to care about those they purport to treat? Unfortunately, such dissent is usually quashed with cries of 'This is what the (financial) providers want'; 'protection of the public and the need for public policy (accountability/panopticism) are needed'. These cries are in effect a veil (and threat of punishment) to prevent other unspoken truths becoming known – the realisation of the oppression of one's subjectivity and subjecthood. Ironically, the end result is that staff as well as patients have limitations set on their liberty and they have no option but to submit to an oppressive order.

12. An example is Carr Gomm community care, where the author worked for a time during his training as a psychoanalytic psychotherapist, which is modelled upon the Lacanian discourse of the master/slave/university. The workers feel themselves to be in the position of the one who knows (or that they are following a higher truth or knowledge such as Supporting People, NICE, *DSM*, etc.), or are forced to adopt the role of the one who knows by management and to follow ludicrous rules and policy that have no real scientific basis. In effect both clients and workers become alienated and are set up to serve the 'system', negating authenticity.

Chapter Two

Into the paradox

Introducing a necessary paradox

Khôra is a philosophical term described in Plato's *Timaeus* (see Derrida, 1997) as a receptacle, a space or an interval. It is neither being nor non-being but an interval between in which the forms were originally held. *Khôra* gives space – a very important idea in relation to psychotherapy and community living. Jacques Derrida (1997) uses *khôra* to name a radical otherness that gives a place for being. He argues that *khôra* defies attempts at naming or applying an *either/or* logical structure or polarity. In other words, the *khôra* is fully other, defies totalisation, and I believe epitomises what it is to be human; that logic cannot fully encompass this domain, and this is where scientific thinking fails in relation to the human sciences, and proliferation of theoretical abstractions of 'mental health' and 'treatment' fall foul. There is no getting away from *khôra*, but you cannot grasp it either.

Derrida's (1997) reading of Plato is, like many commentators believe, a correct reading in comparison to the logocentric use of Plato's philosophy; that is, readings of Plato which pick out the demonstrably true or false claims, making these the centre of the argument while sending everything else off to the periphery as mere rhetoric or ornamentation; letting logic lead the letter. Derrida argues that the result of a logocentric hegemony of Plato's philosophy and logocentric scientistic viewing of the world (as the philosopher Paul Feyerabend would agree) is that any text (oral or written) is neutralised, numbed, inhibited, even though these heterogeneous forces continue to stir in their inhibited form. The result is that a sanitised version of reality is constructed through the logocentric viewpoint, but something lies still stirring that defies the logocentrism. This is radical stuff, but a radicalism that should be welcomed. As Feyerabend states:

> Proliferation of theories is beneficial for science, while uniformity impairs its critical power. Uniformity also endangers the free development of the individual.
>
> (Feyerabend, 1975, p. 24)

The above statement, like the visceral feeling of reading one of Plato's dialogues, creates the sensation of the opening of the proverbial can of worms. One can feel the decentring of the logocentric viewpoint. It also shows how uniformity, however well intentioned, banishes autonomy and critical thinking; there is no one truth, or even there is no truth, and the person who dares to speak the truth must question their truth-making.

We arrive here at a very interesting point, a point which is crucial to the idea of communities: if a prevailing logocentrism prevails in a certain community, what room for a different reading of the text is allowed? More importantly, if, for example, a law is handed down from government, advising what one should do with 'mentally ill' people, how many readings of truth are banished? This is a very serious question and it is applicable to all parts of human living, not just with regards to communities, but also to the practice of psychotherapy and the treatment of those deemed mentally ill.

Søren Kierkegaard, who was heavily influenced by Plato, describes the logocentric situation that is very pertinent to any talk about treatment of those in mental distress. Kierkegaard writes, in his chapter entitled 'The Absolute Paradox: A metaphysical caprice', from his book *Philosophical Fragments*:

> The thinker without a paradox is like a lover without feeling: a paltry mediocrity.
> (Kierkegaard, 1975, p. 46)

In other words, to live a human life without the acknowledgement of the mystery, the mystical unknown that is at the limits of language (and reason), leads us into a mediocrity of existence. I realise that many might baulk at this statement. However, Kierkegaard goes to on to describe how reason in actual fact seeks a collision: a realisation of the limits of reason. This is the supreme paradox: that all thought is the attempt to discover something that thought cannot think. What is this unknown that reason collides with? Kierkegaard called it the God, others call it the unconscious or the Real – we can never fully understand this. But Kierkegaard puts it like this: how should reason be able to understand what is absolutely different from itself? Reason-mongers who want psychotherapy and mental distress packaged and formulaic have not grasped this, but taking heed of Kierkegaard's wisdom, perhaps one should not even grasp.

Put another way, reason desires its own downfall because reason can never pin down everything, especially when it comes down to problems of the human soul, psyche, or how to live a good life. Kierkegaard called this the consciousness of sin, when one realises the paradox that reason cannot solve everything. It is self-love, or vanity, that thinks reason can be called upon to dominate the world. This self-love shrinks from the paradox; it is offended, because it perceives itself as passive. Self-love is intent on concealing passivity. The offended consciousness or self-love, Kierkegaard argues, can be taken as proof of the validity of the paradox. One truly learns when one is faced with the paradox, self-love dies, the absurdity of many things in life is realised, and one can move on from the *stuckness* that the vicious circle of reasoning has got one into.

Many patients and psychotherapists know this place (if one can call it a place). These are the moments of movement, the Zen moments of realisation, when the panic over the abyss of uncertainty ends, that there is nothing really to worry about (but if there is something to worry about, it is fine to worry, although one may not stop the forces of nature by worrying). It is truly other, new, becoming (not predetermined), playful, and cannot be scripted beforehand. One has to take risks in getting there. As Laing rightly believed, one has to take one's chances with the other sat opposite one in the consulting room; the therapist with the patient, the patient with the therapist. And perhaps what we can take from this wisdom is that living in a PA house necessitates that one takes one's chances with fellow residents, therapists and vice versa. And Laing wrote (which could easily be applied to the experience of living in a PA household):

> True, in the enterprise of psychotherapy there are regularities, even institutional structures, pervading the sequence, rhythm and tempo of the therapeutic situation viewed as a process, and these can and should be studied with scientific objectivity. But the really decisive moments in psychotherapy, as every patient or therapist who has ever experienced them knows, are unpredictable, unique, unforgettable, always unrepeatable, and often indescribable. Does this mean that psychotherapy must be a pseudo-esoteric cult? No. We must continue to struggle through our confusion to insist on being human.
>
> (Laing, 1967, p. 47)

These ideas of Laing again highlight the difficulties of the use of a 'scientific method' and subsequent theorising on how to go about relating what it is to live in a PA house. Do I present the narratives of certain individuals, draw upon themes (as in certain qualitative analyses) and conclude with a general theory? Should I present psychometric measures with mean scores of 'mental wellness' of participants before and after their stay in a PA house? Would this be of any use? I dare to argue that it would not be of much use. Let me explain why.

Chapter Three

Method: In search of an anti-method

The problem of scientific method

Wittgenstein famously ended his *Tractatus Logico-Philosophicus* with the phrase:

> What we cannot speak about we must pass over in silence.
> (Wittgenstein, 1961, p. 74)

To many social scientists in search of a method for scientific study this sentence puts a real spanner in the works. This is because there is much of what constitutes being human that cannot be captured within the domain of the psychological sciences as it cannot be grasped in any way by objective scientific methods: hypothesis setting, experimentation, testing for validity, reliability, repeatability etc.

Martin Buber describes beautifully why scientific method detracts from the essence of the lived human being and violates humanity:

> By its very nature, the eternal You cannot become an It; because by its very nature it cannot be placed within measure and limit, not even within the measure of the immeasurable and the limit of the unlimited; because by its very nature it cannot be grasped as a sum of qualities, not even as an infinite sum of qualities that have been raised to transcendence; because it is not to be found either in or outside the world; because it cannot be experienced; because it cannot be thought; because we transgress it, against that which has being, if we say: 'I believe that he is' – 'he' is still a metaphor, while 'you' is not.
> (Buber, 1970, p. 160)

In the above passage, Buber is highlighting the subtle danger that a scientistic research outlook condemns humans to a false totalisation which results in a separation between the scientific observer and the observed. This position is a fallacy because in reality, in a psychotherapeutic context, there is no separation and thus the observer (or other person) makes up the context in which developed meaning is made. This brings us to the wonderful Scottish philosopher of scientific psychology, John Macmurray (underestimated and little known, but known to the tradition of R.D. Laing).[1] His ideas shed much light in regard to the pitfalls and problems of the scientific method in relation to the human sciences, especially psychological research. I will now discuss some of his ideas from his wonderful book *The Boundaries of Science: A Study in the Philosophy of Psychology* (Macmurray, 1939), which are pertinent and crucial to my task.

The philosophical psychology of John Macmurray: The myth of progress

Macmurray argues that the psychotherapeutic researcher in search of the A + B + C = D or sequential and teleological therapeutic process, bound by predetermined laws, makes the mistake of believing that he or she witnesses or observes the process without affecting this process by their presence; and that this process can be fixed in language by things like psychic entities that are measurable or stated quantitatively or qualitatively.

The psychological researcher believes that in researching human beings and behaviour he or she alone is above being a variable in the research. However, scientific research is also a kind of behaviour so the researcher is not immune or lord over the domain they believe they are objectively observing (Macmurray, 1939). As Macmurray describes, science is a tool that has been created by modern society to solve problems. The need to find a solution ultimately determines the effort to produce science. However, this in turn necessitates changes in social habits and social structures which are demanded in the production of science if such an endeavour is to be successful. In other words, the pressures which determine the production of scientific knowledge determine the development of modern society, and also determine the relation between the development of science and the development of society. Therefore, the results of any scientific research project, no matter how value-free and objective its researchers claim it to be, is very much influenced on a micro and macro level by the actual practice of doing the research.

Macmurray (1939, p. 21) argues that 'A scientific theory is never a fact, but the interpretation of facts in the light of a hypothesis.' In other words, the scientific process is the unending revision of beliefs. The result of this is that science can have nothing to do with beliefs that are not predisposed to revision. Much of so-called scientific psychological research into psychotherapeutic practices and processes is turned into dogma (e.g., the Lord Layard utopian cognitive behavioural therapy (CBT) model of happiness; Layard, 2006). Such a dogmatic, politically fuelled abuse of the results of scientific research actually removes theory from the field of genuine scientific investigation (Feyerabend, 1975). When this happens to scientific theory, we are offending against science and becoming obscurantist. Application of such scientific beliefs (or dogma) is not therefore scientific. Scientists may hold beliefs about the world or about human beings, but they should not be regarded as conclusions about human life and how to live it, never mind dogmatically held up as utopian procedures and implemented at a political and economic level to eradicate human *dis-ease* or mental distress. Such a situation reflects in one sense scientific prejudice: the result of a limited way of seeing the world; a Newtonian scientific methodological outlook. Indeed as Macmurray (1939) argues, such scientific beliefs are perhaps less trustworthy than the philosophical prejudices of the average layman. Prejudices are not necessarily untrue; such prejudices are merely uncritical.

The co-development of psychological science and mathematics and statistics is another area where Macmurray (1939) believes human life has been directly affected by the scientistic 'look'. In advanced Western capitalist societies (and in their evolution) the capitalist framework rests upon the development of mathematical and statistical techniques to control and predict human behaviour in relation to economic development. The practical effort towards new modes of life in such societies depends much upon science but as well on mathematical and statistical measurability. Therefore, the large-scale production of commodities (and people are commodities as per Lord Layard's CBT back-to-work psycho-policies; Layard, 2006) for individual countries and the worldwide market can only be possible if the qualitative value of production and goods (e.g., psychotherapy services and treatments, patient outcome, returning to work, earning, spending capital) can be measured by a common and universal standard (e.g., *DSM* diagnosis of depression; reduction in negative automatic thoughts in depression by 12 sessions of CBT as measured by the Beck Depression Inventory; back-to-work figures; see Beck, 1967, 1976; Beck, Steer, & Brown, 1996; *DSM-5*, APA, 2013).

The very serious stumbling block that psychology and psychological research has – especially in psychotherapeutic research – is that if psychology is a science of human behaviour, then there must be a psychology of psychological research. Psychology itself is an example of human behaviour, and thus any general theory of human behaviour must be applicable to every kind of human behaviour, including the behaviour of the psychologist (or researcher investigating psychotherapeutic effectiveness) (Macmurray, 1939).

If the psychologists can give a scientific account of their own behaviour in producing psychological research, they must consider their behaviour as a process or processes which occur in accordance with objective laws. This unfortunately means that the idea of their theory being true or false is excluded. By making their behaviour the focus of psychological research (or the study of the psychology of psychological research) they have made it impossible to regard it as an activity informed by an intention of which might be correct or incorrect. From a scientific vantage point, a scientific theory is simply a belief held by a certain number of people. A scientific account of such a belief would show that people who hold such beliefs, under the conditions of obtaining such beliefs, could not hold any other beliefs. By demonstrating this, it would also show why certain other people refuse to accept these beliefs and could not do anything but reject them. Therefore, the paradoxical conclusion is that the psychologist's account of psychology, if it is to be scientific, must exclude the possibility of considering it either true or false. This depicts a human being as an automaton; by taking a strictly scientific standpoint, the psychology of psychology ignores, because it is unobservable, the possibility of a person's intention or volition. Such a theory is obliged to treat another human being involved in any human activity as just facts that occur as a result of behaviour predetermined by psychic laws that result in someone carrying out an activity and holding a belief compared to another person carrying out another activity and holding another kind of belief.

Of course, humans do have intentions, can hold co-existing beliefs, can carry out activities that they know are wrong, bad, good, misguided, and can make an effort to change their beliefs and behaviour. The point is that to regard human behaviour as under the cosh of universal laws creates the idea of volition as being illusory. This highlights the limitations of psychological science and brings up the important point that there are forms of knowledge which are not scientific. If psychological science were the only true form of knowledge about how to live a human life, then unfortunately psychological science and the practical application of such science would be gravely mistaken; doing psychology is only one kind of behaviour and one kind of knowledge amongst many others; it may help some people, but it may not help others, some may like it, others may not.

At this stage in the history of psychological science and the knowledge that such an activity produces, it must be asked why such knowledge is being used as the gold standard in thinking about mental distress. It is a serious question; what fuels the desire for psychological theories and their application above the use of other kinds of 'knowledge'?

Macmurray (1939) argues that the motive underlying the drive and use of psychological science is, amongst other things, the desire for progress. This has not changed since Macmurray's time; our modern culture and society is filled with the discourse of psychological progress in the guise of psychopharmacology for shyness and overactive children, the development of cognitive techniques online to think more positively, to the proliferation of the phenomena of life coaches. Now the presence of such a desire for progress presupposes that human beings are dissatisfied with their psychological state. In other words, the widespread use of applied psychological knowledge in the realm of mental distress is because we are dissatisfied with ourselves. How this dissatisfaction has come about is a complex issue. Human life since the beginning of time has been accompanied by dissatisfaction. However, different cultures in our time and in other times (for thousands of years) have got along quite well without psychological science and the other modern professions concerned with mental health. As touched on above, Macmurray outlines one reason for the drive for progress of psychological science: the development of psychological science determines the course of societal development, and societal development affects the development of psychological science. Psychology determines what makes someone happy; society takes this on board as 'truth' and finds that it is not quite satisfied with its happiness levels (as distress will always be about); and consequently society demands of science to come up with better theories of happiness. A vicious circle ensues. Of course in other cultures (past and present), viewing distress as something to be eradicated, cured, treated is not something they would consider, yet they seem to get along quite fine (see Kingsley, 1999; Kalweit, 1987; Meier, 2003, for example). And of course, capitalistic culture has the effect of demanding psychological distress being 'accounted for' to a greater and greater degree; commoditisation makes the world go round.

However, the argument that we as human beings are dissatisfied with the status quo and thus demand progress to counter the plight of mental distress is very ambiguous. This could mean I am dissatisfied with myself and you with yourself. Or it might mean that I am dissatisfied with you and you with me. Either of these versions may fuel the desire for a scientific psychology. However, the effort to achieve a scientific psychology will be different in both cases. The state of mind in which I feel I need to comprehend my behaviour is very different psychologically speaking from the state of mind in which I feel the need to understand the behaviour of other people, would you not agree? The need to understand my behaviour or psychology will surely arise from the desire to control and alter my behaviour and psychology. However, and this is getting very serious, the need to understand other people's behaviour can arise from the desire to control and alter their activities. In the second case mentioned above, I may be quite happy with myself and have no desire to change myself. Macmurray (1939) argues that the most direct way in which the desire to control other people's behaviour can arise is when I can see that unless I can control the behaviour of other people, I will be forced to change my behaviour against my own volition. It is this state of mind where one desires knowledge of other people which may correspond most closely to the identity of scientific psychology. The psychologist is the observer (or researcher) of other people. The corresponding practical attitude is one in which the psychologist deems herself to be the agent and the people under observation to be instruments (under the cosh of predetermined laws or forces). Macmurray (1939) suggests that the psychological condition for the production of psychological knowledge is to be found in a mindset where individuals are conscious that their own lives are being frustrated and their purposes rendered ineffective by the behaviour of other people over whom they have very little control. This state of mind gives rise to an effort to acquire knowledge to enable one to control other people's conduct. If Macmurray's thesis is correct, for the development of scientific psychology (as well as allied professions dealing with mental distress) as a social movement and phenomena at this time in history, there must be a widespread feeling in society that our lives are unsatisfactory and that the way other people behave is responsible for this. Macmurray argues that if we blamed ourselves rather than other people for our dissatisfaction with life, the result would not be the great drive we see today for a scientific bias in controlling our psychologies, but rather a religious movement on a large scale or at least something akin to such a thing.

Scientific psychological experimentation (and application of psychological treatment) has been called 'controlled observation'. If such a method is introduced into human psychology and behaviour this must mean that human behaviour must be observed under controlled conditions. This in turn must imply that the human behaviour (or psyche) under observation or treatment must be under control. If one is to control a person's behaviour for the purpose of scientific research or treatment, this person must be what the researcher or doctor/therapist wants him to be and not have his behaviour or psyche determined by his own intentions. The person under such observation must either be unconscious that the researcher/doctor/therapist is controlling him or he must consent to it. If he consents to it, he subordinates his will to the researcher/doctor/therapist and takes orders from her. In either case the person under observation becomes an instrument for the researcher/doctor/therapist for accomplishing her scientific intentions (Macmurray, 1939).

All of what is written above may sound like a very far-fetched Orwellian scenario. However, it is not so far-fetched if one considers events in the near past and very ominous present. I am of course referring to the backlash against institutional psychiatry in the 1960s (see Cooper, 1978; Mullan, 1995; Laing, 1967) and today's anxious drive for progress and war against and cure of mental distress (which is regarded, wrongly, as mental illness) in the guise of: CBT via the government's Improving Access to Psychological Therapies scheme; NICE guidelines for depression (see www.nice.org.uk); *DSM* (e.g., *DSM-5* (APA, 2013), the fifth edition, with even more mental disorders added since the last edition); the misguided and failed attempt by the Health and Care Professions Council's statutory regulation of psychotherapists and counsellors; and the recent Professional Standards Authority policy (assured voluntary regulation) to try to regulate the talking therapies. Such a control system with such sub-systems and their respective ideological discourses does indeed conform to Macmurray's (1939) warnings of letting psychological science infiltrate the very way we see our lives and how we live them.

I now want to turn to the origins (or perhaps a critique) of Western thought – primarily as an introduction, through the philosophy of Parmenides to begin with, which will offer more fuel for thought (or for the un-thought) and which hopefully will explain why an anti-method is a more fitting tribute and account of life inside a PA house and the people who have lived there.

The origins of Western thought: An alternative way of seeing ourselves, of living and 're-search', contra the medico-scientific psychological gaze[2]

I hope to find a way of conjuring the atmosphere of what the praxis of a PA community house is like; an atmosphere where the ground under our feet is never static, at times non-foundational, where perspectives are continually moving, moving to a point, and then moving again, which resembles how a human being's life is actually led; life not as a static entity (e.g., personality, ego, identity) but as breath. I believe that if we take the idea of the human as a static identity as fact, we are creating a fiction or phantom that usurps our humanness. In other cultures (e.g., ancient Greece) this mode of thinking was not the case (see Heidegger, 1962).

I want also to explore the idea of the *Other*[3] in Levinasian terms which fits nicely with the idea of non-foundational or static identity, especially so in psychological research terms. For if I am to pursue the anti-method in this present study, consideration of the *Other*, and a non-totalisation of the *Other*, is a must for research and for healing; a point the psycho-technicians, psycho-bureaucrats and regulators seem to forget so easily. Closely related to this is the idea of health. Too many of us proclaim what health or mental health is for another person or group of people without realising that such prescribing is actually unhealthy – a fine paradox indeed.

Parmenides, Heidegger and Levinas: The problem of psychologism, Being, and the *Other*

Parmenides was purportedly a philosopher born approximately 2,500 years ago who introduced the concept of logic to the Western world. Recent archaeological evidence suggests he was more than a philosopher who was the founder of Western logic, but also a kind of priest, healer, or even shaman. Often people regard Plato, who lived 100 years after Parmenides, as the king of philosophy, and cite Western philosophy as being just a series of footnotes to Plato. Yet, it is now argued that Plato was very much influenced by Parmenidean thought (Kingsley, 1999, 2003). The debates go on about the role and philosophy of Parmenides (there is not the space here to consider them), but a whole host of continental philosophers and psychoanalysts have been influenced by Parmenides including Heidegger (1998), Levinas (1998, 2007), and Lacan (2007) for example.

Charles Stein (1995) sums up very succinctly the Western dilemma contaminating the Western scientific outlook, using the philosophy of Parmenides. In a close reading of Parmenides' poem, parts of which have survived in 19 fragments, Stein shows the anti-cybernetic[4] stance taken by Parmenides in relation to being and relating as human beings (the cybernetic stance is prevalent in psycho-technological thinking in scientific research today). Under the title of 'Phantom Ideality', summarising Parmenides' poem, Stein writes:

1. Ideality is a mode of appearance, of 'seeming-to-be'. It is the mode of the phantom. It arises under a variety of conditions: sensuous, conceptual, intuitional, constructional, and so forth.
2. The reality of a phantom is the undecidability of the reality of a phantom. (A ghost that does not tease belief is not a ghost at all.)
3. Whereas a perception reports of an entity that seems to be, a phantom shows an entity whose being can neither be confidently asserted nor denied.
4. In truth, all perceptions and all determinate thoughts share this phantomatic character, but do not seem to do so. In the phantom the true relation between being and appearance, for a moment, and, as it were, under a veil, shows itself.
5. The ideality of the sign, the ideal signified, is a phantom. Upon close inspection, we cannot decide whether the signified is reducible to the class of the sign's references, or, irreducible, points to an 'ideal object' in a universe of signifieds, an ontological zone unique to the ontology of signs.
6. The objectivity of the world and its temporally extended objects is a phantom, a world of phantoms. We can neither admit nor

> deny the independence of the 'things' from their constitution in our consciousness, our history, our culture.
> 7. The objects of mathematics, when we consider the indeterminability of the great foundational systems – classical, intuitionist, formalist – are phantoms. We cannot decide without dispute regarding their ontological status. They resist final determination as mental constructs, social conventions, or independently existent entities.
> 8. And the temporal present – the famous 'now' point – is phantomatic. It determines that which in our experience is most concrete; it serves as a limit, in fact, for the experience of concreteness: there is nothing more concrete than the unmediated present instant; whatever is most concrete, takes place 'now'. And yet, in itself, the present cannot be grasped but as a 'cut' dividing two other phantoms, the future and the past. It situates the unique, and yet it is perfectly generic, there being no difference between one 'now' moment and another apart from the phantasmagoria of their evanescent content.
>
> (Stein, 1995, pp. 18–20)

Stein's schemata of 'Being' taken from the wisdom of Parmenides' poem helps loosen the bonds and knots of the technological stance fraught with misleading psychologisms, and brings us to what Heidegger described beautifully in the introduction to his book *Being and Time*, referring to the necessity of restating the question of Being:

> This question has today been forgotten ... Not only that. On the basis of the Greeks' initial contributions towards an Interpretation of Being, a dogma has been developed which not only declares the question about the meaning of Being to be superfluous, but sanctions its complete neglect. It is said that 'Being' is the most universal and the easiest of concepts. As such it resists every attempt at definition ... In this way, that which the ancient philosophers found continually disturbing and self-evident such that if anyone continues to ask about it he is charged with an error of method ... the 'universality' of 'Being' is not that of a class or genus ... Thus we cannot apply to Being the concept of 'definition' as presented in traditional logic, which itself has its foundations in ancient ontology and which, within certain limits, provides a quite justifiable way of defining 'entities'. The indefinability of Being does not eliminate the question of its meaning; it demands that we look that question in the face.
>
> (Heidegger, 1962, pp. 2–4)

What the wisdom of Parmenides and Heidegger teaches us, especially in relation to this present study, is that 'inventing' psychologisms, psyche entities, conceptual ideas of being, and the trustworthiness of our signs (language) is quite phantomic and that these strategies do not lend themselves to a truly 'scientific' theory of *Being* This presents problems for both process- and product-orientated teleological psycho-scientific researchers. The most obvious one is that if one cannot define an 'entity' of the psyche for example, one cannot measure it, account for it, or trace its development from one time point to another. Further, one cannot make meaningful comparisons of such entities from one person to another, yet alone at the end of the research process formulate a theory for replication based upon such 'entities'. Such entities are not static in time, do not lend themselves to scientific or mathematical conceptual nature; there will always be 'slippage' or something will be missed when applying scientific and mathematical criteria to people. If this is the case, we are left in a very precarious position, or are we?

It should be quite clear at this point that the standard psycho-scientific methodological approaches which most psycho-technicians take for granted, whether they are quantitative or qualitative, are not value-free or objective, and might well be applying unnecessary and misleading totalisations to people under the guise of scientific research. Of course I am not saying that all scientific research is negative,[5] but when it comes to the issue of mental distress, psychotherapy, and how people live their lives, such methodological tools are not as sharp as one might like to think. This is where philosophical reflection plays its part (and should play a part within an anti-method), or to put it more succinctly as Heidegger (2001) advocates, we should look at this question in the face. This does not imply that we cannot attain meaning or insight by not adopting such scientific methodology. It also does not mean that we should think more; we should perhaps again take Heidegger at his word and actually think less, or at least only think in the methodological sense when we actually need to, instead of blindly going down a research path without really considering what we are doing.

Heidegger was acutely aware of the problems of metaphysics and human beings being thought of as the rational animal (see Heidegger's *Zollikon Seminars*, 2001). Animality is therefore considered from this point of view, from rationality, as being irrational, and thus without reason; interpreted against the 'human intellect' as what is instinctual. From this state of affairs and from the study of metaphysics and its scientific repercussions, the result is that the mystery of living and *Being* is ignored or neglected. In such a scenario human beings under the cosh of a psycho-scientific agenda are exposed and interpreted under the guise of neurochemistry or psychology (i.e., cognitive theories of mental functioning and psychopharmacology within the UK's National Health Service). Both neurochemistry and psychology presume to seek the riddles of life. However, Heidegger argues that such strategies will never solve the riddles of life because science adheres only to the penultimate and must presuppose the ultimate as first; searching for facts, final causes, and conceivable truths which adhere to scientific principles, which in return banishes mystery and the forever unknowable that gets away as a result of using such strategies (Heidegger, 2001).

It has been said by some that poets are probably on to a better thing pertaining to concerns of the soul, suffering, and the mystery of being, and that poets and poetic thinking is more apt for healing our mental distress. I think Heidegger (1971) would agree to the latter as he subscribed to the notion of letting mystery *be* and arguing that thinking is not knowing, but perhaps it is more essential than knowing because it is closer to Being in the closeness which is concealed from afar. Truth, he would argue, dwells in everything that comes to presence; it (presence) is the essence of all essence. Therefore to experience this is the destiny of the primordial thinker. The thinker who thinks or experiences like this knows in essentiality the essence of truth (not just the essence of the true) as the truth of the essence (Heidegger, 1998).

And we cannot focus purely on our own research interests or purely on the problem of being an individual; we exist with others; there is always the *Other* to consider; an *Other* that is often and tragically thrown to one side by the psycho-technician researchers. As Purcell aptly argues, in favour of not forgetting the *Other* in research, drawing on the philosophy of Levinas:

> Methodology stands under the aegis of alterity. If as Levinas says, 'philosophy is the wisdom of love in the service of love', then it will always be summoned to go beyond its current confinement and extend its endeavours to render an account of the relationship with the Other to the Other ... The Other is a question, the answer to which is always inadequate. Methodology is thus subverted in two ways: it can only proceed dialogically, as Rahner might term it, and diachronically, as Levinas indicates. Because the subject matter of philosophy is a relationship between self and the Other[6] who is excessive with regard to the self, but whose very excess will sustain the relationship, the Same and the Other can neither be said in the same time or the same place. Thus, methodology finds itself robbed of a stable ground which would provide a sure footing for its transparency.
>
> (Purcell, 1998, p. 56)

Indeed Levinas, drawing on Platonic ideas such as 'the Good' or 'the *Khôra*', went beyond 'Being' or ontology, as a primary focus on ontology or Being commits a violence to the *otherwise* than Being or beyond Being

– the beyond Being, which shows itself in the said (or the logos, reason) in an enigmatic way, but is always betrayed. Beyond Being has a resistance to assemblage, the presence of manifestation, contemporaneousness, conjunction, and conjuncture. This beyond Being, showing itself enigmatically, signifies the diachrony of responsibility for the *Other*.

Diachrony is an enigma; it is the infinite and does not become a meaning of Being; responsibility for the *Other* comes first before ontological concerns, before representations of Being, before logos, before reason, before synchrony (Levinas, 1998). Diachrony is a non-linear, non-teleological, non-synchronic regressive idea of time in which ego or self does not attach ontological meaning or essence to the *Other* (person or persons). It is transcendence from a linear regressive movement (or progressive movement) along temporal series; parting from a synchronic structure. A simple example of a synchronic structuring would be the extrapolation from memories and attributing the *Other* with an essence of some kind, or some kind of projection into the future based upon ideas of essence (e.g., predicting depression or positing that somebody is at risk for depression). A diachronic structure (if one can call it a structure) grants the *Other* freedom whereas a linear and synchronic attributive stance towards the *Other* would close freedom off (i.e., diagnosing somebody with a mental illness based upon questionable or limited criteria). What we need, to combat the synchronisable time and the violent said as a result of the totalising said or logos, is the force of scepticism inherent in diachronic practice (Levinas, 1998).

Western philosophy, Western psycho-technicians, and the state[7] refute diachrony and associated scepticism with their discourse of the said, of what is 'Being', of ontology, and their egoic logos. This stance is a refutation of any kind of transcendence from this totalisation. The logos, as Levinas eloquently states:

> ... has the last word dominating all meaning, the word of the end, the very possibility of the ultimate and the result. Nothing can interrupt it. Every contestation and interruption of this power of discourse is at once related and invested by this discourse. It thus recommences as soon as one interrupts it. In the logos said and written, it survives the death of the interlocutors that state it, and assures the continuity of culture ... it is in the association with philosophy with the State and with medicine that the break-up of discourse is surmounted. The interlocutor that does not yield to logic is threatened with prison or the asylum [or cognitive behavioural therapy by the government if one is out of work][8] or undergoes the prestige of the master and the medication of the doctor ... The discourse then recuperates its meaning by repression or mediation, by just violences, on the verge of the possible injustice where repressive justice is exercised.

> It is through the state that reason and knowledge are force and efficacity. But the State does not irrevocably discount folly, not even the intervals of folly. It does not untie the knots, but cuts them. The said thematizes the interrupted dialogue or the dialogue delayed by silences, failure or delirium, but the intervals are not recuperated. Does not the discourse that suppresses the interruptions by relating them maintain the discontinuity under the knots with which the thread is tied again?
>
> (Levinas, 1998, p. 169)

From the wisdom of Levinas, we can take heed more clearly of the problems of today's psycho-medico-scientific research into mental distress and this present exploration into the PA communities. There is no room (in the state) for silence, intervals (for not doing), doubt, mystery, diachronic time, the *not* said, and for the unthematised. Because of the productive nature of mental health (e.g., targets must be met, efficiency must be shown) there is little room for an alternative way of 'being with' mental distress. Indeed, in university research departments, quotas of publications are needed to secure departmental funding and even individual jobs. Such a system cuts the knots of ethical freedom for individuals in mental distress to experience the knots as they are, to be silent, to do nothing, to wait, and to rest.

People often find themselves in life under the cosh of violent totalisations where they cannot move freely and develop how they choose to. Everything from depression to schizophrenic-type disorders may very well be the result of stifling totalisations wrapped in the blanket of synchronic time and the pressure to solve 'riddles' through scientific logic (the new God) of how to live. Such people are, it seems, under a spell to capture and reify notions of entities, identities, and use shallow thoughtless psychologism through the use of language, but they don't realise the limits of language and how they are alienated from language; the Real, in Lacanian terms, always abounds.

Sadly, it seems that many of today's psycho-technicians and researchers have turned their back on Plato, Parmenides, and their modern-day advocates. Their God is logos and they feel that this is the only knowledge.[9] Yet, as I have already said, scientific knowledge and methodology is only one kind of knowledge and methodology amongst many others. There are other routes to health and healing apart from the results of scientific research and knowledge. I believe that the Philadelphia Association and the ethos of their community houses recognise this important distinction and make it realised within their community houses. And it is important in the context of this study to recognise this. If I were to present a theory in culmination of this present research project, this theory could be taken by others wanting to capitalise on it; to apply it as a tool on others in another context. But if such a thing were to occur, then the praxis of what I intend to show has occurred in people's lives living in the PA houses would be lost. The scientific discourse would cut the knots, the intervals, and the silences of the lives of the people who kindly agreed to be involved in this research.

What occurs (or at least is attempted, but not always completely successfully) in the Philadelphia Association community households is nothing more mysterious than trying to let other people be and find their own voice and health in their own time. Each story and each individual is different and to generalise to other people and contexts as if this is the formula would be a very precarious business. From a scientific point of view such generalisations would be meaningless. One would (in the present study) need to take into account so many variables that it would be impossible for replication. One would have to consider time periods, personal histories, length of stay, medication, demographics, type and number of residents in house, the house therapists and their training etc. I could go on, but as the reader can hopefully see, the scientistic hope of proving a scientific account of what I will present is that such an endeavour would be very unscientific, and very stupid. Of course, there may be aspects of the praxis of living in a PA house that can be ascertained and considered thoughtfully, but at the end of the day, each individual has to find their own individual healing praxis; this includes therapist, researcher, and resident of a community household. The problem is one cannot really think one's way out of one's problems, and one cannot gain or regain good mental health like one regains good physical health from the application of medicine. That is the great myth that the psycho-technicians want to sell the public: one can get good mental health and one can be cured of mental illness. This leads us to the problematic of health.

The problem of health[10]

In the realm of physical medicine, illness can be fairly well defined; some say the same about mental distress or mental illness. However, with both physicality and mental faculties, the concept of health is enigmatic. As Heaton (1998) points out, health cannot be produced (or predicted or coerced I may add) by means of a technique, whereas some illnesses can be eliminated by medical techniques. Techniques depend on the application of rules to get to a fixed end point or goal. Health in the realm of mental distress is not a fixed goal but is unique to the individual: spontaneous balance. Thus, in the realm of mental distress, therapeutic action involves responsible action (or the ability to respond responsibly; the individual has to find their own ground here within and in considering the social world), and therefore, cannot be reduced to a technical procedure. Each 'case' is a unique experiment so to speak: unreplicable, unrepeatable, and only valid for each individual person; therefore, scientific extrapolation flirts with error at every turn and is infected with value judgements as to what is right/wrong, good/bad, acceptable/non-acceptable. This highlights the problem of technical or productive reason versus practical reason.

This is not a new problem. This problem was discussed by Aristotle in his *Nicomachean Ethics* (see Dunne, 1993, for a comprehensive review of Aristotle's ideas on health, technique and praxis etc.). The difference between technical dealings (or productive dealings; *poiesis*) with mental distress versus practical reason (*praxis*) is that in technical dealings (including research and treatment) the object is to produce a work or result and we use techniques to produce this result. In such productive sciences, the rules for producing the object or goal are apart from its instantiation; the object is to produce a work or result apart from the doing and making. In other words, a doctor may use antibiotics to get rid of an infection, or a surgeon may know how to fit an artificial knee in a person, but this does not necessarily lead to health. An example closer to home is how the clinical psychologist may know 'a theory' of positive cognitive restructuring and teach it to a depressed patient. However, such a method does not necessarily lead to better mental health; a patient may know the theory by heart, but it may have no impact on his or her mental distress. Indeed, the clinical psychologist with her theory of cognition has a far greater handicap than the surgeon who specialises in artificial knees; the surgeon knows intimately the workings of the artificial knee as he can measure it and observe it. The clinical psychologist on the other hand cannot measure cognition as one measures an object, because cognition is nowhere – it is not an object that is measurable or observable like the artificial knee (Wittgenstein, 1980; Heaton, 1998, 2010).

Returning to the idea of the practical sciences or *praxis*, this way of working has its rules only in the tradition of their application, instantiation or interpretation. For example, with mental distress, the rules by means of which one reaches an end cannot be known as objects in abstraction, as with physical medicine (e.g., turning negative cognition into positive cognition in CBT compared to fitting an artificial knee); with regards mental distress, one cannot extricate the individual from his or her lived situation, or for that matter extricate the therapist(s) from their role in the praxis of the situation with the person suffering mental distress. In the situation of praxis, one knows the 'rules' only in a very limited way within the tradition of their application (i.e., silent meditation is needed for Zen monks to achieve *Satori*, but there is far more to it than that; indeed, the monk may have to stop silent meditation for a while to achieve *Satori*).

In the situation of *praxis*, one is not concerned with the right choice of means for a given end, but with finding and realising the end we desire. *Praxis* is therefore is not a matter of the mere application of rules but rather realising living possibilities. This needs practical wisdom (*phronesis*; to be minded) which cannot be methodically taught as are techniques requiring inventiveness (*deinotes*) (Heaton, 1998).

Now, *phronesis* or practical wisdom does play a part in the 'treatment' of mental distress, but in our modern age it is getting pushed out in favour of a more technological approach (i.e., CBT, and the IAPT programme in the UK). There is a pressing need for researchers, scientists, psychotherapists, and psychologists to see the necessity of *phronesis* as opposed to a purely technical approach to dealing with mental distress. As Heaton (1998) points out, *phronesis* denotes the ability to respond (to oneself, others, the environment) in a desirable way in the course of living one's life. Therefore, *phronesis* is not a static scientific concept that can be taught as a technique; one can only find one's way in the field, so to speak. *Deinotes*, on the other hand, is just mere cleverness or the ability to master possibilities. This means for someone to be able to act without any sense of responsibility and turn any situation to their profit. In psychology, the psychologist offering strategies or experiments for positive social advantage for a patient (getting people to like themselves and others to like the patient) uses *deinotes* (Heaton, 1998).

However, the concept of *phronesis* is intrinsic to the idea of what it is to be a human with common sense. Therefore, common sense confirms such ordinary things such as when one recognises suffering in another person. It is not the same as a common belief, for example, when a Labour supporter expresses to his Labour colleague that it would be a disaster if the Conservative party wins the general election. The Labour supporter's belief may be common within the Labour party, but not within supporters of other political parties.

The person who uses the wisdom of *phronesis* deliberates about how to live life and is in touch with the vitality of life, a life which Heaton points out has no limit to the kinds of vitality one can choose. This vitality is lived and thus cannot be taught as a technical knowledge; technical knowledge is abstracted from life, and although part of human life, it is not embodied life. Therefore, although technical knowledge can be demonstrated, it is only from the outside of embodied life that it is shown (Heaton, 1998).

The wisdom of *phronesis*, contrary to technical knowledge, is concerned with responsibility (or the ability to respond) to what needs to be done from moment to moment in a lived and embodied human existence: in the *here and now*. As practical wisdom is about responding appropriately, with 'response-ability', it stands in contrast to technical knowledge which does not require *phronesis*. For example, if someone has a certain disease such as malaria, the doctor just administers the medicine that will treat the malaria. Practical wisdom is not required in such an instance. One just follows the biological rules of malaria (Heaton, 1998).

However, a responsible decision can never be completely turned into a technical application such as the previous example. As Derrida (1995) argues, the activation of responsibility will always occur before and beyond any theoretical thematic decision. Responsibility is implicated in singularity or within the individual, as an individual can only be responsible within their own history, knowledge and finitude. Such a responsibility also demands that a person is accountable to the social world – other people. But if this is the case then there must be some kind of thematisation in being responsible. However, to subordinate responsibility under the hammer of objective or technical knowledge is to discard responsibility. As Heaton points out, a responsible decision is made through the confrontation of undecidability, beyond knowledge and of being certain. The thematisation of responsibility always comes up short, but it must be like this – unthematisable. If it was not like this, we would then do away with responsibility and thereafter become irresponsible (Heaton, 1998).

Scientific research aims to be objective and serve in every context just like scientific research into depressive cognitive schemata aims to be universally applicable to human beings. The research into depressive cognitive schemata can be repeated and verified by other cognitive psychologists, and any variance from the general theory of cognitive schemata can be accounted for by more research. The technology of cognitive behavioural therapy is the application of the results of research into depressive cognitive schemata. But the application of CBT depends upon standardising its technology as much as possible: to control and objectify. This fixed goal, the objective and controlled application of the technology of CBT, becomes a monadic entity. However, such a fixed goal, as Heaton (1998, 2010) eloquently puts it, is very different from the varying goals of practical reason and what it is to lead a human and desirable life. Human life is in a context of constant change and the person in it is part of this context and so the whole context shifts with time and in different contexts and with different people.

These flaws of empirico-cognitivism cast some doubts over the whole cognitive revolution in relation to mental health. However, as Wittgenstein so beautifully put it, there are even greater dangers of being seduced by empirico-cognitivism and derivatives from this and the related psychotherapies and mental health treatments relying upon models of the healthy mind:

> You observe your own mental happenings. How? By introspection. But if you observe, i.e., if you go about to observe your own mental

happenings [as is done in CBT; noticing negative automatic thoughts] you alter them and create new ones and the whole point of observing is that you should not do this – observing is supposed to be just the thing that avoids this. Then the science of mental phenomena [cognitive schemata inherent in the theory of CBT][11] has this puzzle: I can't observe the mental phenomena of others and I can't observe my own, in the proper sense of 'observe'. So where are we?

(Wittgenstein, in Monk, 1990, p. 500)

Wittgenstein would answer in response to this last question that we would be in a fog of confusion that cannot be resolved by an accumulation of more research or data on cognitive schemata in depression and how to cure depression. Neither can this confusion be resolved by a new theory of cognitive schemata. The only thing capable of clearing the fog is a conceptual investigation (i.e., the concept of negative automatic thoughts; 'I feel unhappy')[12] which shows that these words gain their meaning from a form of life (i.e., a language game). This is very different from describing, explaining and scientifically researching physical phenomena (Monk, 1990).

Thus, in contrast to the technical and scientific application of cognitive techniques, which rely upon a notion of some immutable human essence (e.g., cognition), *phronesis* or practical wisdom depends on the historical nature of man (the man in his lived and embodied experience) rather than an ideal and absolutist system or theory pertaining to the cognitive function for example. Our knowledge about ourselves is not scientific knowledge. Therefore, as Wittgenstein (1980) argues, it is futile to have a scientific account of the mind, as where is the mind? We cannot measure it, we cannot see it, and we cannot do anything to it resembling the scientific research as is done in engineering, for example.

As Heaton points out, people are very easily deceived by the perceptual metaphor of introspection. He argues that people confuse the ability to say how things are with us, what we feel, what we think, or what we are wanting, with our ability to know and perceive. Thus if somebody says to another person, 'I am angry with you', the person is describing how they feel angry with another person, not describing how they perceive anger in themselves. This is not a report of what the person knows; it is an emphatic assertion, not the result of an investigation. This point takes us back to the issue of responsibility. For a person to express what they feel or think, they must respond appropriately to the situation and their place in this context. This is in contrast to a technical or scientific way of responding. The application of a technological way of dealing with or responding to the situation (for this person) is dependent on the technology, rather than being aware of their responses to their context (Heaton, 1998).

It is helpful here to return to Plato (in Cooper, 1997) to remind us that there are two different kinds of measure. Plato urges us to distinguish *metron* from *metrion*. *Metron* is between measure and what is measured. This involves standardised values and a mean, mode, variance, and standard deviation etc. *Metrion* is what is fitting or appropriate. One cannot impose a measurement as one does on an object in *metrion*. A *measured action* would be an example of using *metrion*. An individual's 'mental health' does not have a measurable standard. Indeed, mental distress or mental health must be differentiated from norms or averages, as norms and averages require standard values.

Healing mental distress takes the emergence of something natural or hidden from view; to become attuned to the world. Therefore, therapy for mental distress is something that is beyond norms, standards and the technological application of rules. Attunement to the world is only found by the individual re-emerging from mental distress (or some kind of hermeneutical transmutation taking place), with the finding of their own feet or rules and standards and recognition of appropriateness and responsibility in their world of others. If the person in mental distress becomes the target for scientific intervention, labelled by abstract norms, and treated technologically, this is irresponsible because the person in distress has to come to find him- or herself *responsible* in the world.

Therapy is derived from the Greek *theraps* meaning service, attendance, or care. The psychotherapist serves or attends to the person in mental distress. This is not a technological approach. This approach involves addressing the person in distress in a responsible way. It requires, as Levinas (1998) argues, recognition of their otherness, and the uniqueness of the person and their situation. It thus cannot be dependent on the application of rules, standards or norms. As Cooper (1978) said, norms impose needs, they do not recognise them. This can be frustrating for the person suffering in the throes of mental distress as they may want a cure based on sound, reliable, scientific principles (as in certain physical disorders) but this is not so simple to achieve with mental distress.[13] Preconceived treatment plans based on *poiesis*, a teleological frame from point A in space and time (e.g., depressed) to point B (e.g., cured, happy post-treatment), is fuelled by the discourse of the master, or even the discourse of the university or hysteric (depending on how one conceptualises what discourses are in operation, as the discourses operate fluidly and are interchangeable within and between individuals) (Lacan, 2007). Dialogue, conversation, or silence, and living amongst others with a telos or meaning of such activity being for the activity itself (not for an idealised end point contaminated with a telos of achievement or production), is such a praxis/*phronesis* which differs from a technical-calculative process/*poiesis* (Heidegger, 2001). A praxial telos used in silence, conversation, or living with others can be used as a way to engage *phronesis,* as opposed to the smothering through technological applications or discourses of oppression concerning the treatment for mental distress. An environment that cultivates *phronesis* requires the ability for people to listen to one another, the capacity to attend to one another, to leave one another alone when needed, but more specifically, the ability to be responsible and to use measured actions rather than irresponsible regulated strategies which discard ethical obligations to others and oneself.

Statement for an anti-method

These (above) are the philosophical reasons why I have been in search of an anti-method in this present study of people's experiences in the PA communities. In this final section of the chapter I want to reiterate 'theoretically' (which is perhaps ironic, in a necessary way, to get to where I am going) why I think it is justified to proceed by way of an anti-method. However, to be fair it was not just an (a)theoretical manoeuvre to get to where I am going: I had to use my confusion and bewilderment to guide me; the usefulness of these will become apparent later. Anyhow, if I am to proceed ethically and responsibly in relation to the material I feel I must continually be mindful of falling into any error – of *not* totalising the state of affairs with which I am confronted.

The unfortunate thing (or perhaps very fortunate thing for the purposes of *discovering,* not *covering*) is that I am going to write about people's suffering, disappointment, anger, loneliness, but most of all struggle. It is this that I cannot get away from and that anyone who understands what I am trying to relate here will understand. There is no hell without heaven, and no heaven without hell; struggle is the key to what I will write about of those who have lived in the PA houses. As one participant told me, those who live in the PA houses walk between two worlds. I take this as a responsible acknowledgement of one's suffering and others' suffering in the world and that this may be a route to finding contentment and peace in this world. It may be that we cannot have one without the other. Levinas's (1998) inspired writing shines a light through or lifts a veil on much of what has gone wrong in our culture of accountability, mastery, and transparency. As mentioned previously, Levinas argues that Western philosophy, Western psycho-technicians, and the state refute a praxial way of living and the associated scepticism with their discourse of the said, of what is 'Being', of ontology and their egoic logos.

Similarly, Foucault (2007), in *The Order of Things,* highlights the danger of order and measurement via logos and rationalisation in the human sciences:

> Measurement enables us to analyse things according to the calculable form of identity and difference.
>
> Order, on the other hand, is established without reference to an exterior unit: 'I can recognize, in effect, what the order is that exists between A and B without considering anything apart from those two outer terms'; one cannot know the order of things 'in their isolate nature', but by discovering that which is the simplest, then which is the next simplest, one can progress inevitably to the most complex things of all. Whereas comparison by measurement requires a division to begin with, then the application of a common unit, here, comparison and order is a simple act which enables us to pass from one term to another then to a third, etc., by means of an 'absolutely uninterrupted' movement. In this way we establish series in which the first term is a nature that we may intuit independently of any other nature; and in which the other terms are established according to increasing differences.
>
> (Foucault, 2007, p. 59)

Therefore, by using either ordering or comparison by measurement, one gleans facts, and the facts depend on what facts one looks for, which obviously omits or excludes facts. As in any ordering or comparison of measurement, one cannot include all the facts. In effect we become blinded by factual taxonomies. This scientistic objective posturing reduces people's lives, experiences, and actions to the logos which, as Levinas (1998) describes, nullifies the gaps, the intervals, the slippage, and recuperates these into the logos. If we are to be honest, the gaps, intervals and slippage do not disappear, but this is where Western scientific method has gone awry by ignoring this.

Feyerabend (1975) would agree with the latter sentence, but goes further in his critique of qualitative research. Drawing on the philosophy of Parmenides, he states:

> ... a theory is inconsistent not with a recondite fact, that can be unearthed with the help of complex equipment and is known to experts only, but with circumstances which are easily noticed and which are familiar to everyone.
>
> The first to my mind, the most important example of an inconsistency of this kind is Parmenides' theory of the unchanging and homogenous one. This theory illustrates a desire that has propelled the western sciences from their inception up to the present time – the desire[14] to find a unity or 'substance' behind the many events that surround us. Today the unity sought is a theory rich enough to produce all the accepted facts and laws; at the time of Parmenides the unity sought was a substance. Thales had proposed water, Heraclitus fire, Anaximander a substance which he called the

> *apeiron* and which could produce all four elements without being identical with a single one of them. Parmenides gave what seems to be an obvious and rather trivial answer; the substance that underlies everything that is is Being. But this trivial answer had surprising consequences. For example, we can assert that (first principle) Being is and that (second principle) Not Being is not. Now consider change and assume it to be fundamental. Then change can only go from Being to Not Being. But according to the second principle Not Being is not, which means that there is no fundamental change. Next, consider difference and assume it to be fundamental. Then the difference can only be between Being and Not Being. But (second principle) Not Being is not and therefore there exist no differences in Being – it is a single, unchanging continuous block. Parmenides knew of course that people, himself included, perceive and accept change and difference; but as his argument had shown that the perceived processes could not be fundamental he had to regard them as merely apparent, or deceptive. This is indeed what he said – thus anticipating all those scientists who contrasted the 'real' world of science with the everyday world of quantities and emotions, declared the latter to be 'mere' appearance and tried to base their arguments on 'objective' experiments and mathematics exclusively. He also anticipated a popular interpretation of the theory of relativity which sees all events and transitions as already prearranged in a four-dimensional continuum, the only change being the (deceptive) journey of consciousness along its world line.
>
> (Feyerabend, 1975, pp. 43–44)

Thus, as Feyerabend shows, experimentation, fact and law gathering do in fact create the idea of change, difference and taxonomy. However, and this is a more accurate reading of Parmenides' ideas, such processes uncovering *Being* and *Not Being* do not fundamentally depict actual facts, as Being *is*, and cannot *not be*. Put simply, our humanness (logos, cognition, rationalisation etc.) is limited and veils Parmenides' 'One'. Thus, when engaged in fact finding in psychological science, we are always one step behind as we cannot really know where we might have gone astray, and we may not be able to pinpoint any theoretical synchrony.

In effect, what madness am I proposing in how I will proceed in trying to decipher interviews of people who have lived in Philadelphia Association community households? I fear I am proposing a *foundationless* exposition which may be regarded, at the very least from logical/empirical, qualitative and quantitative methodological vantage points, as *non-sense*. Indeed in many ways I am proposing a foundationless exposition, or more accurately, I feel I may be giving much-needed space to the often covered-over diachrony as Levinas might say (Levinas, 2007). But there is a method (towards an anti-method) in my madness I believe. This is as good as any an idea to end on and proceed onward to the following chapters where hopefully such an anti-method becomes clearer.

In the next chapter (Chapter 4) I will briefly discuss the practicalities of how I carried out the research. This will be followed by the individual interviews (edited transcripts) of ex-residents of the PA communities (Chapters 5–18). There will then follow Chapter 19 outlining a schema of how I analysed (or approached) the interviews (how I came to find a gestalt/non-gestalt of sorts within the interviews, their themes and categories that they yielded), and how I found a standard methodological approach incompatible in practice. This will be followed by Chapter 20, which is a more in-depth discussion of the interviews, which expands on Chapter 19. Chapter 21 concludes by offering my final thoughts on this study and its wider implications.

Endnotes

1. John Macmurray is not very well known in academic psychology circles. Indeed, he is never mentioned in the standard UK university psychology degree syllabus, which is a great pity because he has much to offer.

2. By 're-search' I am implying that what I am attempting to do in finding an anti-method for this study is to bring to the surface a mode of being ('being' in a non-foundational Derridean or Levinasian sense) that was once commonplace (i.e., ancient Greece around 2,500 years ago), and is present in Sufi cultures of today, and thus was and is known. Therefore this is nothing new, but perhaps forgotten, neglected, or is not learned today by the psycho-technicians and their patients.

3. *Other*, in italics with capitalisation, is an inference to another person emphasising the importance, in the Levinasian sense, of the other person (see Levinas, 2007).

4. Cybernetic refers to the idea Heidegger has with regards the problem of technology, thought, and human relating; language and information passing to each *Other* in the form of signs which pass as the reality of which Being is based upon. Heidegger saw the danger in viewing Being in such a way and wrote that such a cybernetic or technological way of living the world was thinking gone astray. Being, Heidegger would argue, is not the exchange of information or news to help us guide our lives. From

his reading of Parmenides, Heidegger would argue that information and news as technological devices to help people to live have their place, but quoting Aristotle, he explains (1962, p. 72) why there is much more to human being or being human than the technological information transfer of how we think of ourselves and *Others:* 'For it is uneducated not to have an eye when it is necessary to look for a proof, and when this is not necessary.'

5. Medical research into curing certain degenerative diseases such as Parkinson's and multiple sclerosis is invaluable.

6. Levinas argued that Heidegger forgot the 'Other' and focused only on Being, the individual, which was one step removed from the 'otherwise than being'.

7. 'State' here refers to such psycho-bureaucratic organisations as NICE, Health and Care Professions Council, Skills for Health, and the governmental favouritism for the dubiously utopian treatment of cognitive behavioural therapy in the guise of Improving Access to Psychological Therapies. All these organisations are involved in a grand totalisation of what mental distress is and how to treat such individuals. They rely upon synchronic time, the said, meaning and logos without letting an 'interval' open where a more ethical diachronic space naturally develops. Their psycho-technical discourse cuts through these potential intervals, which are never recuperated, as the discourse is 'forced' upon the populace dressed in the Lacanian dialectic of the master–slave.

8. These are my comments in brackets. This refers to the British government's policy created in 2010 of giving CBT to people who are out of work. This move essentially says to the unemployed: being out of work is the fault of your negative cognitions; science has proved this; we have people to give it to you, thus cure you of your negative brain patterns. No mention is made of course of a poor economic situation, dull post-industrial-era jobs in call centres (the new factories), and the ravaging damage caused by an overly capitalist and materialistic society where narcissistic traits are inculcated into the populace through the media, school, university, and the workplace.

9. I am not against logos per se. Logos is very important and needed. One only has to read the dialogues of Plato to see the value of logos in getting one to the place where one can ascertain the limitations of logos.

10. I am indebted to the work and the ideas of John Heaton of the Philadelphia Association for my thoughts in this section.
11. Author's comments in brackets as an example in relation to the modern mental health care system in the UK.
12. I agree that cognitive therapists investigate with their patients why it is that they feel unhappy and try to deconstruct this with them. However, I mean here to deconstruct the notion of a negative automatic thought. The dichotomy inherent within CBT of negative and positive thoughts sets up an artificial dichotomy. This is paradoxical as CBT rests upon the strategy of getting rid of dichotomous thinking. For example, I would question why negative thinking is assumed as *negative* and positive thinking assumed as *positive*. This assumption rests upon the assumptions of the Lacanian master–slave dialectic (Lacan, 2007): the therapist as master, the patient as slave. Further, it is of dubious scientific validity to judge whether the thoughts of another person are either too negative or positive. More serious though is the idea that one can observe one's thoughts; as Wittgenstein points out, as soon as you observe them, your thoughts are transformed. You can thus never grasp them, as the act of trying to grasp them makes them ungraspable. I would say that the best form of CBT, which many therapists use very effectively, is based upon practical wisdom or *phronesis*, not on a science of cognitive schemata, and therefore not based on a scientific method.
13. Foucault, in *The Order of Things* (2007), describes in detail how language has developed over time (the symbolic) where abstract representation of the world (i.e., mental health) has given rise to a divorce from the world and experience commonly known in other times. For example, 2,500 years ago in the temples of Apollo and Asclepius in ancient Greece there was no such 'grasping' after a cure for mental torment. In a practice called *incubation*, people would go down and give up hope of any change and let healing occur (if indeed it did occur) by forces not under their control. One may call this force God or the Divine, it does not matter. A force was operating beyond human agency that was tapped into. This shamanic practice filtered into esoteric Christianity (e.g., St John of the Cross, *The Dark Night of the Soul*, 2003) and Sufi practice (see Rumi, 1994). This is still practised today. See Kingsley (1999, 2003) and Meier (2003) for descriptions of incubation in ancient Greece. I am grateful to Noel Cobb for introducing and teaching the idea of incubation to me.

14. I must add that I think this is a mistaken desire or incorrect reading of Parmenides' philosophy. From my reading of Parmenides' esoteric philosophy, it is clear that discovering unity via facts and laws was not Parmenides' desire; his ideas were a critique against the possibility of discovering facts and laws through human rationalisation. Thus the idea behind Parmenides' 'one' was not to be of some use in discovering laws and facts, but in the unveiling of an *Other* (be that divinity, God, etc.), where only in the darkness of silence a non-human reason would emerge, guide man, because despite all the reasoning and gathering of facts and laws, *Being is* beyond the grasp of ratiocination, or the signifier, which falsely solidifies ideas and goes against *Being is* (see Geldard, 2007, *Parmenides and the Way of Truth*).

Chapter Four

Practicalities of carrying out the research

Data collection

As a result of the anti-institutional and anti-bureaucratic ethos of the PA houses and how they are/have been run, record keeping has not been a major priority. Some phone numbers and addresses were given to me by the Philadelphia Association from surviving records, and ex-residents were contacted via these means. Other forms of recruitment involved word of mouth and advertising on the Internet on the PA website and the Kingsley Hall website.

Interviews

Most of the interviews (11) were conducted face to face in people's homes, a quiet public place (e.g., cafe), or at the Philadelphia Association headquarters in Hampstead, London. Two interviewees were sent a pro-forma questionnaire (see Appendix) – a guide outlining key themes which I asked them to comment on, in as many words as possible or as they felt they needed. There was also a section inviting interviewees to write about anything else if they so wished. The two people I sent questionnaires to sent them back to me via email and through the post. One other interviewee recorded his answers to the questionnaire on an audio CD which he then sent to me.

During the face-to-face interviews, I used the pro-forma questions only as a guide to ascertain and make sure I covered key information about the houses which was pertinent to the study (i.e., the positive and negative experiences of the houses, how somebody got accepted to live in a PA house etc.).

All interviewees were informed about the study at the first point of contact, and again when a meeting took place. They were informed of the nature of the study and that I was researching the experiences of ex-residents who had lived in one of the PA community households. They were informed that the results may be published in some form but that all personal identifying data and characteristics would be taken out.

Twelve of the interviews were transcribed, verbatim, by hand and typed up and made into a Word document. The other two interviews were typed and/or written into a Word document by the interviewees (i.e., written answers in response to pro-forma questionnaire). The Word documents of each interview were sent back to each interviewee to check that they were happy with the record of the interview (and their answers) and if they wanted to make any amendments. If they wanted to make amendments, these were included in the new (amended) Word document for analysis. The interviews contained within this book are edited to the extent that the material pertaining to the residents' stay is included as much as possible, where material judged not related to the study is excluded for reasons of confidentiality and in trying to be concise to the material I wanted to convey in relation to the study. The text guide for the reader when reading the interviews goes as follows:

Italics: The speech of the ex-resident.

Non-italic font: Bruce Scott [BS], my speech during the interview.

Bold: My comments that have been written as part of the analysis – my initial thoughts and comments. These were not part of the interview that occurred.

(Italics): This indicates information that was said by the interviewee, but has been anonymised for the sake of publication. All other anonymised information (i.e., dates, ages, towns, names of countries and people etc. are self-explanatory and shown within the text by either arbitrary letters, *A*, *C*, *Y*, *X*, *XX*, or numbers (i.e., Therapist *1*, *2*, *3* etc.). Some fictional names have been created to help the flow of the text in places.

[Non-italics]: Further clarification for the reader, but not actually said by the interviewee.

Interviewees' characteristics

Fourteen people were included in this study. There were seven males and seven females. The age range of interviewees was between 28 and 75 years old. All but one was a native English speaker. The interviewees stayed in PA communities over a wide range of times and places: Kingsley Hall (1965–1970), Archway (1970–1979), Portland Road (1971–1980), The Grove (1972–present), Ascot Farm, Stadhampton (1977–1988), Shirland Road (1983–2006), and Freegrove Road (1996–present). All these community houses worked/work in different ways, and had/have different therapists and different ways of meeting (e.g., amounts of house meetings if any).

All of the interviewees could be described as having experienced some form of mental distress which was *one* motivating factor for them to end up living in a PA house. Many put into question what their distress meant to them in relation to their life experience; it would be fair to say that for some, living in a PA community was as much a political move as it was for the benefit of their *distress*. I say this in the Sartrean sense (Sartre, 1972) of making one's illness or distress a weapon as a force of agency to escape oppression from malevolent forces (i.e., psychiatric hospital, psychiatric drugs, institutional mental health care). Three out of the 14 interviewees (after leaving their PA household) take either a low-dosage psychiatric medication or very occasionally, in times of stress, some kind of tranquilliser when needed. Two people approximately once or twice a year visit a doctor or psychiatrist for a check-up for their own peace of mind. Two people have needed a psychiatric hospital stay since leaving/finishing their PA community house/stay.

As far as I have been able, I have kept names, dates, places and personalising details anonymous.

Part 2

Tales of *Docta Ignorantia*: Interviews with ex-residents

Do not give up, then, but labour at it till you feel desire. For the first time you do it, you will find only darkness, and as it were a cloud of unknowing, you do not know what, except that you feel in your will a naked purpose towards God. Whatever you do, this darkness and this cloud are between you and your God, and hold you back from seeing him clearly by the light of understanding in your reason and from experiencing him in the sweetness of love in your feelings. And so prepare to remain in this darkness as long as you can, always begging for him you love; for if you are ever to feel or see him, so far as is possible in this life, it must be in this cloud and this darkness. And if you are willing to labour eagerly as I tell you, I trust in his mercy that you will reach your goal.

(*The Cloud of Unknowing*, Anon., 2001, p. 22)

Chapter Five

Diana

Bruce (BS): How did you find out about the houses?

Diana: *I was in (another establishment) and I became friendly with a former resident and when it became time to leave (this other establishment) ... I thought I would try to move into a PA house. I decided, vowed that when I left the centre that I would not go back to how it was. It cost me blood, sweat and tears to achieve that* [her state of 'wellness'] *... so the PA seemed the next logical step to ensuring that that did not happen. So it was word of mouth. I don't think I would ever have heard about it otherwise.*

BS: So it was not really publicised [the PA houses]?

Diana: *No, not at all. I don't think it is publicised anywhere near enough ... Had someone when I was 18 said to me you can go somewhere to live where your housing benefit will cover it, you can take your dog and it won't be an issue, my life would have been on track a lot sooner and that's a bit frightening.* [When she was younger] *I had no support. Oh, they thought, hospital staff, I was just attention seeking so I had to up the ante to prove I was not attention seeking, that I did need it and that I did need help. And then you get in a vicious circle. I am quite angry about the institutions I have been in. I have been in too many hospitals and I have been sectioned too many times and I have been locked up on locked wards too many times, secure units, because people just did not understand how I dealt with things ... it's why I think the PA should fight to keep the houses going. I think they need to do a lot more work and I think particularly things should change a little bit and people should be aware of what it is actually like to live there and be more honest. There is no us and them ... of course there is an us and them ... you're there as a resident with issues, your therapist comes in and you know ... Acknowledge there is an us and them. That does not mean someone is superior or better. It acknowledges in fact there is a difference. Living in the houses can be extremely stressful at times and at times there is not enough support in the PA houses. I mean you're trying to work through your own shit and then you also have to deal with everyone else's shit.*

BS: So it can be chaotic?

Diana: *It can be incredibly chaotic ... And the downside of therapy is it is always looking at the negative ... very little congratulation, you're doing really well, it's great ... but there is no space in a house meeting for that ... there is no time. You know ... three hours a week is very little to go actually go on ... and that is not enough time ... if you have three or four people that are having a shit week that's not enough time to work out what is going on. The other downside is that all the therapists never see what is actually happening in the meetings, which in my experience is entirely different from what is actually going on.*

BS: So in some sense, were the house meetings a censored version of what was really going on in the house?

Diana: *It's like looking into a Petri dish. All you see is what is under your nose. You don't actually see what the bacteria came from or anything that makes it up ... and that gets missed and I think that's crucial. I think there should be more casual input* [social engagement from house therapists] *... not just the house meetings ... It made a difference and other residents said it made a difference. It was nice to see the therapists as human. It was nice to have something else other than what's in the house meetings which is often the worst of people, or the best of people, depending on what they are bringing. So I think that is a bit of a shame. There is not enough one-on-one with the house therapists.*

The conversation then moved on to the topic of Diana's experience of psychiatric hospital.

Diana: *There were a couple of good staff ... they were not overrun* [with patients there]. *You have got two to three staff per patient. It's a better ratio and some of the staff will only do it and because it's quite highly paid. A couple of those were on their way to do psychotherapy training. So they were very much more open and you know, the crazies that were there were completely off this planet ... For the first few years no male member of staff would sit alone in a room with me because* [hospital policy] ... *When I first went into hospital I was suicidal. I tried to take my own life approximately three or four times a year. I have played Russian roulette. I am lucky I have dodged many, many bullets ... I don't actually know how. So then to go somewhere where they were attempting to do things differently, it made a huge, huge difference. I think sometimes some people who go into the communities don't have the capacity. They have not hit rock bottom with the psychiatric services.*

BS: Do you mean the people who go into the PA communities who have not hit rock bottom?

Diana: *Yes ... some people have, some have not* [hit rock bottom]. *And I think generally ... if you have not hit rock bottom or if you haven't seen what the world has to offer in terms of support, you can't value what's different and you still might fight and kick against it but that's part of the process and I guess that's why I went in vowing I was going to make a difference ... that I didn't want to continue my life like this ... you know life was pretty shit and the world doesn't ... I mean even now it's bullshit ... people say there is more openness to people that have or has had mental health problems and that's crap ... and the PA houses do make an effort to normalise. I always describe myself as acting quite normally to an abnormal situation. The house almost follows that philosophy and that people are there for a good reason. That should be more in hospitals.*

BS: Do you mean the reason that people become distressed is because the situations they have been living in beforehand have been chaotic and contributed to the reason why they are there? I mean, if you get upset at another guest it's not your illness, how the psychiatric system might view it, it's just part of life.

Diana: *To some degree yeah, I think. I don't think that this was always remembered, that everybody is human and I guess ... you kind of need people* [in the house] *that are semi-sorted, you need people that are at least certain that they want to get sorted and it makes it difficult when you are living in a house and people kind of want to, but they don't really understand what it entails. They don't understand therapy, they don't understand that actually the houses are going to be hell, but you have to want to make a difference in your life and that's when it becomes difficult and the house is fractured in that sense. It's very hard. You always have people at different stages but you have to have people at the same starting point ... which is: I am going to make a difference to my life for real. As we experienced in our house, too many people moved in and left, loads of people didn't even make it a year ... you know one person who left too soon than she should have managed to actually stand and say goodbye to us. Maybe that was as much our fault as theirs, but I don't think it is about blame but those people I think should have been somewhere else. They should have been more supported.*

BS: Are you saying that these kinds of people didn't see that the house was not some kind of hostel?

Diana: *No they didn't. They didn't have their eyes open to how difficult it was going to be ... when I got into therapy, I did not have a clue. You know, after three months friends from back home asked are you feeling any better, has it worked, and I said to them it does not work that way, you know it's an ongoing process but I think when you are in therapy you get to a point when you realise actually you are the person who is going to make a difference, yes you need support, you need people around you, but only you can make the difference. If you are still expecting everybody else to fix you and you go into a community where pretty much everybody else is struggling to sort their own stuff out, they are never going to be able to help anyone else unless you are helping yourself. They feel let down because they don't feel supported.*

The issue of too much therapy or the oppressive 'therapeutic nature' of the PA houses was discussed.

Diana: *I think it should be made compulsory for everyone to take a holiday. To get away from the house ... you need to get away from everybody, you need to take time, you need to do things as a community, but you need to feel you have your own breathing space ... in the back of everybody's mind, these are the therapists – they are going to be analysing ... it's not surprising that people lock themselves in their rooms and don't want to come out and don't engage with people ... I certainly did at the end of the day. I did once, I did shut myself in my room and watch TV ... I did not want to have to deal with other people's shit ... I did not want to have to share my shit with other people ... I just wanted to switch off ... I just really wanted to have space. But having said that, give me a community any day of the week rather than a hospital, and that's the thing people don't realise ... however bad it might be in a community, it's bad for the right reasons ... how bad it is in hospital, it's bad for all the wrong reasons. You know, you get drugged up, you have side effects. I was given a drug that gave me all the side effects* [symptoms] *that I had before, before I was given the drugs in the first place which is never a good thing.*

Diana discussed that since her stay in the PA house she had virtually come off all psychiatric drugs but that she saw a place for them – not a cure, but as a form of self-management when she needed to take them (a point she emphasised several times during the interview). The importance of individual therapy was also expressed.

Diana: *I still take sleeping tablets and diazepam p.r.n. ... when I need them ... When I went to the (another institution before her stay in the PA house) I was on depot injections, tranquillisers, really heavy-duty sleeping drugs. The list was as long as your arm and they all had side effects. I still hallucinate. I fortunately don't hear voices, but I see things all the time. The more stressed I get, the more hallucinations I get. I manage them and I manage them well and nobody has a clue that this is part of my life and I've had to deal with it and it's the one thing I disagree with ... I feel that this is now part of my life and I have to manage it. I don't think they are ever going to go away. I would give anything for that to happen but that's how my brain reacts when I get stressed. It never used to and if I never spent so much time on drugs and hospital perhaps it never would have done. But if I manage my tiredness levels, if I make sure I sleep, if I am not sleeping, then I know that I need to take some sleeping tablets for a couple of nights. Because if I can manage that and occasionally if my anxieties get out of hand, if I can manage that before it gets to a point then I have been able to reduce going back on the harder drugs; its self-management. You know I have been drug-free for three to four months, and then I can have a stressful couple of months but I guess because I am aware of the side effects, I manage quite well ... but I suppose that's the therapy as well. It helps with that. Drugs do have a place don't get me wrong, I hate the damn things, they have a place when someone ... I mean I've had a suicide in the house ... My own personal opinion is that drugs only work if you've got people working alongside you. Sometimes it needs both. Most of the time the thing that actually makes a difference is the people, having someone to understand, having someone to talk through stuff with, having someone letting you know in the middle of a panic attack that you are not going to die ... OK you might be afraid you are but you know, I am here, you are going to get through this.*

BS: In regards to the house, how were drugs viewed in the house?

Diana: *Anti ... very anti ... the drugs ... and I kind of agree with it and it's only kind of later I have revised my views that it has its place. Having said that I would have never come off my drugs and I don't think people who have not been on heavy-duty drugs ... no one is going to know what it is actually like, how it can fuddle your brain, and the fear that you might need to go back on them and it is one of the things, personally I watch my symptoms very carefully. I know my warning signs and I try to avoid them. Touch wood I have only needed to go back on antipsychotic drugs for a short period once in the last four years and that was for a couple of months and I was able to come off them again ... I want good services, I don't want people who are going to put me straight on drugs or going to dismiss me or just use my label and not realise there is a human being underneath. That's where the houses work. Labels, they don't hold much weight. It's sometimes useful to know. For me, when a hospital is giving a label it's just to let someone [know] what they are dealing with ... It's to make everybody else happy ... you need to know it in some ways ... so the houses work in that sense.*

BS: Were you encouraged to get into your therapy apart from the house meetings with the two therapists?

Diana: *You have to have your individual therapy; I kind of think that is crucial. There are times in the house, I think pretty much everybody feels this at some point ... you feel completely got at by everybody else ... and you need to know that somebody is on your side and your side alone. It's weird, I think the houses almost play out ... they play out the family groups, sibling rivalry, the arguments you know ... so you kind of need to go through all of that. You need to feel as if everybody is getting at you at some point. It was only after when I had left the house that I was able to reflect and realise myself, that if I had actually volunteered to take the blame for something that actually I wasn't being blamed at all. I was jumping in way before ... and if I had just shut the fuck up it would have went to whoever the therapists were referring to*

The need for other activities, other than house meetings, was voiced by Diana.

Diana: *I don't think there has been a house trip. So you need something else. Whatever it might be art therapy, garden work etc. . . . you know something that caters to the other side of the holistic view ... talking is not always the answer. Talking can often lead to conflict, upset and fear whereas if you are actually working or painting or doing something ... I mean you are never going to please everybody but I do think it is too much talk and not enough engaging with people on a different level. I feel you need different support and I think the houses could improve greatly if they could recognise that talking, while it's great, but if you're not in a space to actually articulate where you are at you need something else to help you through that period ... and maybe in our house some of the people wouldn't have left if there was something going on. Maybe they would. It's quite worrying too many people in our house moved in and then moved out too quickly and that made it certainly ... made me ... and I know some of my other housemates feel like failures; what were we doing wrong, between ourselves.*

As discussed before in Chapter 1, there is no time limit placed on residents' stay in PA houses.

Diana: *When something is open-ended no one is going to ... you know you have got to do something pretty drastic to get kicked out ... it can make people lazy. On the other hand some people need that to come to and stay and you know they want something different. It's difficult, it's a double-edged sword, it can work both ways. I think, I know they have the, 'where is it going?' chat, with you but I think it needs to be a little bit harder you know, we have had people live there and not use house meetings and that can be very frustrating and I have been through periods where I bowed out of house meetings ... and you kind of need that balance. Yes you need to be able to rebel for a bit, but if it goes on for too long ...*

This took the conversation on to the issue of 'the shock' for someone moving into a PA house and getting used to the routine.

BS: So I suppose if all you have had is a hospital ward experience, coming to a PA house must be quite a shock?

Diana: *Yeah, but moving into the house is a shock even if you are used to therapy ... it can be a terrible shock to move in ... and you know we had one lass move in, she had never done housework one day in her life. She was expected to partake of a rota. It's a tall order. You have got to grow up quick ... it's a shock and I don't think there is enough ... I don't know ... I wonder now in retrospect whether some of the people ... if they had had just a little bit more one-to-one support in the beginning, someone, one of the therapists or a student or someone that just could help them ... I mean you try as hard as you can as residents but you are dealing with your own shit ... you have got your own triangles going on with your housemates or your therapist and it's very hard to always be aware of someone's mood and actually it raises issues and people don't always get their head round it. I can remember someone arguing coming out of a house meeting going, 'I don't get it ... it was just a damn light bulb ... I did not change it, what's the big deal?' ... and I was just sitting there thinking no, that will just come to you if you stick at this long enough, it takes a while to get used to that and kind of you have to find your own way, but the communities are intense ...*

... the breaks [when the house therapists are on holiday] *are a big shellshock, you don't have any external help, people generally tend to act out, their therapist has gone away, the house meetings have stopped, the structure has ended ... of what there was anyway ... it's the time when you need therapy more ...*

so just something to bring people together, sometimes the only time we as a house came together was during the house meeting, if you were lucky ...

... You learn most when it is difficult and I think that's why I think a break from it, a reward, a pat on the back ... you have done well at this ... just something that is needed for you to stick at it. I think it is unfair to expect people to move in and live in hell. There is nobody in their right mind would move in to one of these houses unless they had to work for something ... because they are difficult and uncomfortable and you have got to be prepared for it, but actually that's what challenges ... it's difficult. People have to find their own way. But it's nice to be given the opportunity to find your own way. But I think it was incredible how many residents would leave, because it was difficult.

The importance of the houses was emphasised by Diana in the role it has had in her recovery. This brought up the paradoxical nature of living in a PA house.

Diana: *If you lose the houses, if you didn't have the houses I wouldn't be a functioning member of society. I would not be working somewhere I feel useful for the first time in my life, I feel like I want to contribute something. I hope it does not sound too negative. It is almost part and parcel; you don't have the houses without negativity. I know I would not be where I was today ... I lived now two years in my flat. For the first time in my life, a two-year period on my own, without being in hospital, without having a major breakdown as it were. Take the houses away and I would still be in a psychiatric hospital. I would still be drugged up ... I would be on benefits with no hope of being any different. For the first time in my life I can actually form relationships. I don't by any means think it's all sorted but I don't think anyone is ever sorted.*

... The PA should not feel bad if they can't meet everybody's needs and in that sense it's not, I have lived with too many people where talking therapy at times is seen as the worst thing in the world because the more you try to get people to talk, the more they shut up, close up and retreat into their distress ... watch Big Brother, they are just like what the communities are like ... look what happens when you put supposedly a group of the members of the public in there, it's all the same conflicts, all the same issues, it's all about community life. Why

would we watch *Big Brother* ... we live it. You put people together who are sane and you end up with intense crazy people. Stick all the members of the PA in a house together for six months, expect them to be completely tolerant and open and sharing when actually people have different ways of living and it does not always mix. It was once said to a resident, a friend of mine, that if she could survive a community she would have no worries about surviving the rest of the world. Yeah, the rest of the world is not as bad as the houses she said. It's a shame the rest of the world does not recognise that's actually a good quality, that actually you can come through hell and you can live in hell.

BS: It's a hard sell, to sell the houses as a hell that is going to be good for you?

Diana: *You have to go through hell to find your way out ... it's your own personal hell, you can tell people it's actually going to happen but it's* [telling them] *not going to make a difference. However, they do need some preparation. I once had a therapist tell me this doesn't happen because most people would not go into it, because some people won't last if they knew the truth of the matter. Then they are not ready for therapy. If they are not ready for individual therapy, then they are not ready for the houses. It works, but it needs to be more realistic or it needs to be thought about more realistically about what it really is. That there are times when it does not work, and that is what sometimes makes it a success and completely unbearable to live in. I've been to hell and back and it was fantastic! The ultimate result is fantastic, but I would never choose to do that journey again. I hope that's been useful.*

Chapter Six

Cara

A place that valued communal living, the work of R.D. Laing, and a 'therapeutic ethos' was one of the reasons for Cara's decision to move into the house.

BS: What was your prime motivation for moving into a PA house?

Cara: *I think I had positive ideas about communal living. (X) had written me a card in which she said that I could live there with my children. I needed somewhere to stay as my landlady needed my room for a relative of hers. I also thought it would be a place where I could get therapy ... I'd read books by Laing. I heard about the egalitarianism of the houses and it sounded lovely.*

But the difficulties of communal living in a PA house proved not to be a utopian environment.

Cara: *Although there were some people who behaved very responsibly and worked hard, one in particular admirably and consistently so, I think too many of us were too selfish and introspective to bond much as a group. We lacked the discipline, clear common ethos and shared rituals that are found in religious communities, which would have given us a strong sense of community. We had a lot of arguments about mess.*

Cara's desire for a 'more spiritual input' into her life became clear when the issue of individual therapy came up in the conversation.

Cara: *I did not have individual therapy but towards the end of our stay there, the*

PA arranged to pay for therapy which we found for ourselves. I saw an educational psychologist who called himself a Jungian. I chose him because Jung was aware of the link between spirituality and health and my schooling had been traumatic. I continued to see him after I left the house until he casually told me he had lost a painting I'd done which had great significance for me ... Looking back, I realise that what I really needed was family therapy for myself and my children to help us heal the wounds of a long separation from which we still haven't recovered.

Nevertheless Cara found her stay helpful in some respects but felt more therapeutic input was needed.

BS: Was it helpful living in the house?

Cara: *I think it was helpful being there and also helpful in getting my children back. It was a lovely setting. One to one, and have the group* [in addition] *would have helped. Someone to confide in would have been helpful.*

BS: Present-day houses have approximately three meetings per week, and one is encouraged to be in therapy.

Cara: *I think that is what is needed, one needs support like that. Also, it is very important to have a high ratio of people who have worked through their problems already living in the houses to prevent us from destroying each other. I am ashamed of some of the hurtful things I said to people under the guise of being honest.*

The conversation then moved on to the topic of psychiatric drugs and her thoughts about psychiatric hospitals.

BS: You were on about the ethos ... you mentioned a *few* people were drinking and smoking cannabis etc. What was the attitude about psychiatric drugs?

Cara: *I am not sure. I don't know if anyone was on psychiatric drugs. I imagine people were there partly because they didn't want to take them as they are so harmful.*

BS: I suppose that leads us on to the topic of psychiatric care.

Cara: *My first experience of being a patient in a psychiatric hospital had been following an overdose of sleeping tablets about 14 years before living in the PA house. I had also had two brief stays following the birth of one of my children seven years after my first admission ... On each occasion I'd taken my own discharge* [from the hospital]; *I can't bear to think of what might have happened to me if I hadn't ... The lack of privacy, bullying, and mystification* [in the psychiatric hospital] *is enough to drive anyone mad let alone the medication and ECT* [electroconvulsive therapy] *or the threat of it.*

BS: So quite harrowing [in reference to her hospital experience]. How do you think your horrific experiences compare to the house you stayed in?

Cara: *Of course it was much, much better* [the house compared to psychiatric care] *even though it was difficult. But unfortunately there was not the support to prevent two of our former housemates, C, an artist, probably diagnosed with bipolar disorder and A, whom I believe had been labelled with schizophrenia, dying in their mid-40s of the effects of major tranquillisers, one in 'care in the community' and the other in the back ward of a mental hospital. By the time C was found dead in his bed in a halfway house, his life had consisted of little more than getting up late, attending various centres for the mentally ill, getting his injections as required, attending to his bodily needs and going to bed very early, he'd long stopped painting or any other form of artistic expression.*

I think A's incarceration and untimely death could have been avoided, had any of the other women in the house, myself included, noticed and befriended her ... 'No man is an island' ... She was quite sensitive and pretty and greatly relieved not to be in hospital. When I visited her on the ward, some time afterwards, I did not recognise her; she looked at least 20 years older and it was hard to follow her speech, which was faint and indistinct. She was dribbling and incontinent and limping, because, since I'd last seen her, she'd leaped from a bridge. I was very distressed at seeing her like that and, to my shame, I reacted in the typical but least helpful way by not going back. I did visit her several times more though. One day, about six weeks before her death, I thought of her and my conscience was troubled at having abandoned her to her fate; I resolved to remedy this as soon as possible. She cried with joy on seeing me and said that she had been praying that I would visit. She wanted to make me a cup of tea but was rudely prevented from doing so by a male attendant, who, when challenged by me, tried to justify his actions by saying that she drank too much coffee. I got my tea but I did not like the way she had been humiliated in front of her guest and wrote to the hospital to complain. The next time I returned, it was with E, an advocate and a member of the Society of Friends with a strong social conscience. When A told us that she was continually being pestered by some of the male patients on the ward, E soon put a stop to the abuse. She also arranged to take her to a drop-in centre for women run by MIND once a week.

We went once and A enjoyed the atmosphere of warmth and sense of freedom to be herself and looked forward to going again – a major step on the long road to independence and rehabilitation. Unfortunately she was unable to travel much further on that road as shortly afterwards she died of pneumonia. The last time I saw A was a few days before her death; she was in a terrible state of health, breathing noisily and with difficulty but allowed to go about the ward insufficiently clad for a cold day. She should have been in a general hospital. The staff were genuinely dismayed at her death. I don't expect it would have occurred to them that the massive doses of antipsychotic medication she had been on would have greatly weakened her immune system and made her unable to fight the infection. As with C, the autopsy report said that she'd died of natural causes. At least there was a strong staff presence at the cremation. Apart from myself, there was no one who'd known her from the PA. The officiating minister spoke of a bright young, sports-loving woman who enjoyed life to the full, sadly struck down by a tragic illness, from which she was never to recover, whilst in the final years of her student nurse training. A life obscured and cut short by a psychiatric history!

BS: Have you any last thoughts you wish to express?

Cara: *I am told that nowadays the PA houses are more structured and supportive and if that is the case I hope that there will be many more of them. I have written at such great lengths about A because had the Philadelphia Association house lived up to its name and provided her with the protection and affirmation of brotherly love that she so desperately needed, you would be able to interview herself. Unfortunately as I had not bothered to attempt to get to know her until it was too late, I can tell you little more than the minister, who had not even met her, but I can leave you with a poem* [see below] *she wrote for the patients' magazine, when an inpatient, before she came to live in the PA house. It reminds me of a saying of a great prophet that God said 'I was a hidden treasure and I desired to be known so I created the universe.'*

Thoughts on the Living World
Pondering on moments
With joy that makes me cry
Up here amid nature's charm
The grasses, bright flowers and a sky so calm,
I think of lonely moments shared,
The fact that we all breathe the same air
Gaze at the same sky, hills and sunshine
and what is yours and mine.
For the World is One
There is peace and hidden treasures for everyone.

Chapter Seven

Roland

Roland is a man who seemed to have had a positive experience of living in the house. He is now working full time and is living in his own flat.

BS: How did you hear about the houses?

Roland: *A MIND advocate suggested that I go into a PA house. This occurred while I was in hospital* [psychiatric hospital]. *She knew it was a therapeutic community. I was given a phone number and I phoned it. I just said that I have been given your number and I would like to come to one your house meetings. I had been told that they had house meetings. So I went along to a meeting completely in the dark and I was also quite ill but did not quite realise it. That's the trickiest thing, I kind of ... you know you often base your decision when you are quite healthy and you decide to do things after you have thought through things quite carefully. But I was not in a state to be like that, so I just literally turned up at this house and this house meeting and I just sat with this group. Because I had been in a therapy group before it did not seem anything completely strange to me. I was like oh ... I have landed in a kind of therapy group. That's basically how I found the house ...*

... So after a couple of visits I got a phone call from somebody ... and she told me that I had been accepted. At that point I couldn't make a decision, I mean it was bizarre, I woke up one morning about 2am and I just got out of bed and I started taking all the books off my bookshelf and piling them up on the floor and then I went to another meeting and again the house therapist asked me if I had decided what I wanted to do yet. And I said I can't decide. I told him about the book incident at 2am in the morning and he said, 'Well you have

made your decision, welcome'. When I moved in I just wanted to carry on as usual and I remember one of the house therapists telling me, 'You can't do that, you are ill', and I said, 'No I am fine', and he said, 'No you are not'.

… Then I moved in and they showed me the room and I thought, 'God … I have never been treated like this in my life.' I was shown this room and it was a hovel. The walls were green and I think the door frame was orange and there were these old curtains hanging from the window and there were stains on the floor from candles. I thought do they think I am a dog or something? They just said, this is your room and it was just a complete and utter pit. I thought I might be ill but I am not living in this state. So I said to them can I have some money, can I have some paint to decorate my room and that's what I did. I immediately started to decorate the bedroom and I turned it into something nice. But I could not believe it at the time; I just thought they could have at least given me a clean room.

Being flung into this situation was distressing for Roland and despite his feelings of depression it seemed to spur him into action, to make his living quarters more comfortable, much to the annoyance of his fellow housemates.

Roland: *I mean I was depressed anyway and it really made me feel as though … I am amazed that I started decorating it. I mean that probably helped me. But then I started decorating the whole house and I became very unpopular because I was not asking anybody. I was just going ahead and doing it.*

After settling into the routine of the PA house and staying there for a couple of years the unusual open-ended stay issue came to the fore, which for Roland was helpful in his recovery. But in some ways this open-ended stay created some confusions about when he should leave; in other words Roland had to come to his own decision about when it was time to leave. Further issues were the dynamics of the house which each resident has to struggle with and which Roland certainly did.

Roland: *… When I moved into the PA house I do remember thinking that* [that he would live there for two years and then move on as he thought a two-year stay would be long enough]. *But after two years I still did feel ready to leave and the house therapist said to me that in order for someone to really benefit from the house then you really need to stay there for about five years. So that kind of took the pressure off... that I thought I was failing. I think I was there about six years when I started saying, you know I think I would like to move out and get my own place and it took about a year for that to happen.*

BS: So the view of the therapist that it could take a long time sounded like there was no cut-off point to your stay ... it was open-ended.

Roland: *Yeah ... it's strange you know. I used to think to myself well, I suppose they could turf me out. I mean basically if I am honest with you, I lived in the house like I would live anywhere else. I was working when I was there, I was studying when I was there, I was going to courses and seminars etc., so in a sense I had a social life and in a way I was living in the house as I would in a shared house. Yet in another way I was living as a kind of patient. I got a bit confused sometimes as to which way to look at it. Sometimes I feel angry that I was there for so long and that nobody pushed me out in a way. Sometimes I think I lived there too long and it was a waste. I do get angry sometimes and wonder why did they let me stay there for so long, why did not somebody put some pressure on me? But then I think, well hang on a second, what was the difference of living there ... I mean the difference that I felt is that there was some kind of structured holiday thing in place ...*

BS: When you say structured holiday, do you mean the house meetings that they had every week?

Roland: *Well I felt safe with the therapists there and I would not have felt safe if the therapists had not been there. What I realised is that one of the things that happened in our house was what some people felt uncomfortable about, I certainly felt uncomfortable about it, was that the house dynamics were not really tackled. There was a lot of envy about it; those people who got away with certain things. One of the things about living in a community or being in a therapy group is experiencing that loneliness of being in that group alone and I often felt very lonely there and very isolated at times because I was depressed as well, but then to have this issue in the house made me feel more lonely.*

Following this I wanted to find what was 'therapeutic' about being in the house.

BS: Back to the structured holiday thing you mentioned: you had these house meetings; you were in a hospital before you arrived in the house … What I am trying to say is, what was the thing that was therapeutic about being in the PA house? What is it that goes on in the house that is therapeutic and also is different from a hospital setting? What is it that you can identify as the process that goes on in the house?

Roland: *I mean, they are really difficult questions. Again I do sometimes wonder if I needed to be in the house … I was living in a shared house with about four or five other people and there were a couple of rather nasty people in there. They were treating me quite badly and it was pointed out to me that every time I went home I came back in quite a bad way, but I felt as though I could not move out of there at the time, for one reason or another. So I was offered my own flat and I think if I had moved in that flat I would have had my own space and gotten well naturally, or I had the other option of moving into the PA house … I just felt safe when I arrived. I know I felt safe there because I felt as though … because the fact that there were therapists coming in I thought well if people do treat me badly and if anything does happen to me then at least I have got a couple of therapists coming in. So I thought they are going to protect me or help me. So that was the kind of structure. Again I had people in the [psychiatric] hospital saying to me we think you have had too much psychotherapy and that actually it would be good for you not to have therapy now. So again there was this kind of … when I was mentioning to people that I was thinking of moving into a therapeutic community, people were saying at the hospital, you have had enough therapy now. It's quite interesting because my therapist at the time said to me that I have told your story, you are ready to finish therapy now and I told him that I still feel absolutely crap.*

Roland told me about his old therapist before he moved into the PA house. He was a 'dogmatic type of therapist' who used diagnostic labels freely. This contrasted greatly with the individual therapy he received after moving into the PA house.

Roland: *I mean I remember one day my old therapist who was a clinical psychologist said to me 'I think you are depressed, let's get the DSM-III', and he was looking under the topic of depression and now when I think about it, I thought hang on a minute, he was performing to me ... it felt like a bit of a performance ... whether you use the DSM or not, it was the way he was flicking through the DSM ... 'Yes, you have got this, you have got this, and this,' he said. He said, 'I think you are depressed you know. I think you should go to your GP and get some antidepressants' ... I mean he is still around now. He still teaches now. I think he is quite a good therapist, but he screwed up with me though.*

BS: So you left this guy, and did the therapists in the PA house kind of encourage you in a different direction to get another therapist?

Roland: *They put me in a different direction and the other thing is that I said that I felt crap and I've been told I had told my whole story and then (a house therapist) put me onto this analyst and the stuff that started flowing and I started coming out with this stuff. It was like having an orgasm and all this stuff started coming out, free association stuff and it felt absolutely wonderful to me.*

Roland then went on to talk about the house therapists. He described them as not being dogmatic or overly coercive with him. More surprising for me and beautifully put by Roland, he mentioned the word love and the role of the house therapists.

Roland: *They* [the house therapists] *certainly did not coerce me in any way. I remember having this sense from (the house therapists) whatever I said, people agreed with. This felt quite new to me because I spent a large part of my life saying things and people disagreeing with me. So I have always assumed that I am wrong and that. So that was the thing about the house; people did agree with me and this was new for me. But then the other thing was that I saw the PA house as just a normal house. Even though the therapists came in we certainly did not have formal group psychotherapy. I mean it did feel more like living in a family. The love that I felt from (the house therapists) ... and when I say love it's kind of just the acceptance ... it was far more powerful on a deeper level than I had experienced before.*

BS: It is very interesting that you use the word love.

Roland: *They were very loving in a sense. Interestingly, the word love was not used that much, but it was more so in the caring form of day-to-day living, which I was not used to. This is interesting because there were a lot of heavy experiences that took place in that house, experiences that I never had before; people becoming ill, psychotically ill, I had never experienced those kinds of scenarios and yet everybody was considered. It was not the person who was ill, the whole house was considered.*

BS: How do you mean the whole house was considered? Was this a crisis or something?

Roland: *Well they would respect someone leaving if they left, they would respect someone staying if they stayed. I suppose that was the main ethos of that as a whole the house had to be taken care of. So if somebody was in the process of wanting to destroy that, then that person is not going to get the focus, just because they are ill, but the whole house has to be kept in faith. It felt a very safe place to live.*

In comparison to the PA house experience, Roland made some interesting remarks regarding his experience of staying in a psychiatric hospital, which was just prior to his stay in the PA house. The psychiatric hospital experience seemed to signal to him the need to be able to go 'down' into his despair.

Roland: *When I did go in* [to the psychiatric hospital] *then I just plummeted into a deep, deep, deep depression. It's almost like some part of me, some magical part of me knew I could only do that if there were other people around keeping an eye on me. I could not do it out in the world. So I went into this deep depression, but no matter what they did, they were trying all these different kinds of antidepressants but they did not work. But I obviously needed to go in there … but … everybody stays away from you when you go into hospital. All the staff go into this office. It's like a glass house. You see all the staff in this glass room, all staying with themselves. They all look terrified to come out of this glass room. And there is you as a patient and there is all these mad people running up and down the ward completely naked and you're thinking, I ought to be in that glass room where they are safe ... it's very strange ... very strange to see people in that situation ... but I mean more or less, they just leave you to yourself. Nobody talks to you; nobody wants to really listen to you. So you are just left to your own devices. They give you something to help you sleep at night ... it's bizarre, bizarre ... Most of the psychiatrists see the patient maybe once all the time they are in there. It's quite bizarre how people want to go in ...*

... There are some really mad people in mental hospitals and I suppose after ... that's where the houses come in because there is something missing [in the hospitals] *there are lots of people that can be helped a lot ... but they don't need to be on a psychiatric ward, they need to be somewhere safe ... The problem is a lot of people don't have that and so where else do they go? So sometimes, they will allow them onto a ward but they don't belong there.*

The conversation then turned to things that Roland found difficult or unhelpful in the house. These things included feeling deskilled or disempowered. But the paradox was he described that one has to become 'helpless' to get well. He also went on to talk about the importance of being in touch with his distress.

Roland: *One of the things that was unhelpful was before I moved into the house I had always been very independent ... I had taken care of my own finances and knew how to take care of myself. So to have somebody who was collecting the rent, opening the bills, paying the bills etc., there was something disempowering about that. I often thought that kind of help did not feel helpful. If I had felt more in control of having to pay my rent, pay my contribution of the gas/electricity, water, it would have felt more natural to me. So I felt like I was being deskilled and of course now that I am living on my own I feel empowered again. But there is another way of looking at it; I always think that therapy is in a way about being in a state of disempowerment you know because I felt more in control before I went into therapy; you have to learn to be vulnerable, you have to learn to lose ... it's all part of getting in touch with our pain and learning to lose. It's often felt like a lesson in disempowerment ... I was living with people who sometimes did not want to cooperate and what I discovered was, it was one thing to be in a therapy group and to have disagreements and disruptions, but then you only see the therapists for a few hours a week but in the house you are there all the time. So if you confront somebody you have got to live with consequences of that. So that was difficult. There were some people there that were using the group scenario to get at you. They would store things up and use the group meetings to get at you. That always was not very helpful.*

BS: How did you get helped with your depression being around all that?

Roland: *That was the point really. Since leaving the house I don't know whether or not I still have depression, and I know people have said to me, you are not depressed. The house therapist was saying I don't think you are going to have problems with depression now. I mean I am very well; I work ... I do all this stuff, I've got friends, I must be OK. I am dealing with stuff, and yet I still think I suffer from depression. I can just feel it in my body, and I think to myself, I know if I went to my GP ... I eat like a trooper, I sleep as soon as I put my head on the pillow, I have a sexual appetite, and I am getting on. I know if I went to my GP they would say you have got no symptoms of depression and yet, there is something in me that feels I am depressed. And I sometimes think it is the depressed position that Freud talks about and it does feel very healthy to me to have this [depression]. So I am not clear but I have always been of the ilk – this life is so fucked up, all the wars, poverty and stuff happening in the world. One should be depressed with all that is going on and I do wonder sometimes, could I have done without the house? I don't know.*

I then asked Roland about his views of the whole experience and whether the PA house experience lived up to his expectations. This part of the conversation highlights the paradox of human life; that distress and misery may just be a necessary part of the human condition that we must all face, for not to face it may cause us to lose our humanity.

BS: The last couple of things. Did the house live up to your expectations and did you get out of it what you thought you were going to get out of it?

Roland: *I don't see myself as a success story as somebody who has left the house. I don't feel that I am a good person to talk to about the houses. OK I have left and I am still struggling, but I guess who is not struggling? So I see somebody like (X)* [an ex-resident of a PA house]; *she is a success. But that might be my biased perception. I have always shared mostly* [lived in shared houses] *and have only lived on my own twice and here for about three years. So I can live on my own but I don't see that as a success story. Often I think I have done all this therapy just to live on my own. It does not seem to make sense. I missed the house when I first moved out and I missed the sense of belonging to a group of people. Coming home there, there was always a sense of something happening. So again when I lived in the house I thought I can't wait till I get my own place and now that I have got my own place I think it would be lovely to be with other people. I have never been able to get my head around the idea that living on your own is something healthy and yet therapeutically speaking they* [therapists, mental health professionals] *say that if you can't live on your own, you can't live with anybody …*

… But I miss the houses and the odd thing is, I have learned to deal with conflict with people and tolerance of people. I also appreciate the fact that people might not like me and not having to do anything about it, whereas in the past I would have gone out of my way to get people to like me.

BS: So you feel more at ease in your skin?

Roland: *I feel more at ease in my skin, but not completely though. I would recommend it* [the houses] *to anybody. I can see how it helped … therapy does work I think.*

Chapter Eight

Joe

Joe is another person who had come upon the PA after his discharge from a psychiatric hospital. He was drawn to the PA as a result of its connections to and the reputation of R.D. Laing. Firstly, Joe spoke warmly of one of his fellow ex-residents/informal resident therapist. It is difficult to exactly locate the roles and functions of people who lived in the early PA houses, of which Joe was a part. Suffice to say, although there were no 'roles', some were there to 'help' out, but their role was not to create an atmosphere of us and them. However, inevitably, as Joe and other interviewees described, this was difficult to achieve in practice. I was struck with the warmth of how Joe talked about people in the house, be they more in the role of patient or therapist. Joe had several 'stints' in several PA houses over a period of several years.

Joe: *He* [a fellow resident/resident therapist] *was fantastic. When I first arrived there something he did so impressed me. He took me to the local police station and he introduced me to the local police. He said to them, 'This is Joe, he is alright but he can be a bit strange. If you see him wandering around the streets shouting at the sky about something or pointing at people don't be alarmed. This is who he is and this is where he lives.'*

And I just thought what a fabulous thing to do.

BS: That was nice of him.

Joe: *He was an immense asset to the whole organisation and a very good poet. I really liked him a lot. A lovely man. It's a shame that we threw him out.*

BS: You threw him out?

Joe: *Yeah. It was a kind of anti-therapy revolt. We threw out (two therapists who were residents) and decided we didn't want any actual therapists living there. I abstained from all this. It was other people and I think they were treated very badly. It was a kind of inmates' revolt. They were told to go and live somewhere else. I can't remember what date that was ... probably a couple of years after I had moved there.*

Joe described how the PA house for him was an escape and asylum from what he thought would have been his home for the rest of his life: the psychiatric hospital.

Joe: *And I was expecting to stay there the rest of my life. I was kind of resigned to it. I asked for ECT and they did give me two shots. I just wanted to know what it was like. After the second one there were complications. I didn't come round for three days. I had had a reaction to the anaesthetic or something. Right, so they said. No more for you. And I was given Stelazine* [an antipsychotic psychiatric drug] *which affected my motor capacity and I became a bit of a shuffler. I was really quite seriously ill ... but I was only young ... I was what ... 18 or 19 and my parents had moved abroad as soon as I became ill. So I did feel a bit like an orphan. So I was very glad to be adopted by the PA house.*

Although Joe had arrived in an environment that was by all intents and purposes critical of psychiatry, today Joe feels that psychiatric medication is invaluable for him. Joe also talked warmly of the care he received from R.D. Laing and the ambience he created; an ambience that would not have been present in any psychiatric hospital during this period, or even in contemporary times. Joe described beautifully an ambience where authentic communal living was being strived for but not necessarily in a structured therapeutic way.

Joe: *But the main difference between then and now, then I didn't take any medication. Now I do. That's the main difference. Without medication I am such a different person. Now I am really very well and pharmacy has come on in leaps and bounds in the last few decades. Modern medication is very good ... very smart. I am on something called Olanzapine which suits me down to the ground. I experience no side effects. I think of it as a pacemaker for my brain. It just keeps my brain moving. In those days without medication I did deteriorate very much and Laing himself was despairing that I would ever come out of it. He called me a deteriorated schizophrenic. He was like a father to me really ...*

... everything was informal but quite a lot Laing would arrive and gather everyone up and we would sit down and eat and bring out large amounts of long-life beer and we would drink those and he would talk to us. I don't remember what he talked about but I was a very attentive listener and it kind of soaked in. But he would talk for hours and it was very therapeutic. He had a wonderful speaking voice and we had meetings like that. But individual therapy ... very few people wanted it and I myself was very suspicious of talking therapies. I did not feel that they could do any possible good at all. So I was quite glad we did not have structured therapy. Most of the time I suppose we were talking or attempting to talk to each other. There was a lot of social activity which would have been therapeutic, but nothing organised ...

... Well yeah, there were meetings sure, but they were very impromptu and unstructured. People would just sit around and try to discuss what on earth was going on.

BS: Do you mean between everyone in the house or ...

Joe: *Between themselves. People really didn't know what was happening. The meeting was the way to try to get some idea of what was happening to them. It was a very strange environment. People really used to use the meetings to get a handle or not on who they were but on what the hell was going on. Why were they in the house, who were these people?*

BS: What was the therapists' role there? What did they do as such?

Joe: *Understanding people and helping people understand themselves if that's what people wanted. If people didn't want that it was OK to just do whatever you wanted to do. They made themselves available 24 hours a day but they did not lay down the law and say 'you must have therapy, you are ill and you must get better.'*

Testimony of experience

The idea of an asylum or escape from the clutches of oppression of the state and its hospitals again came up in the conversation.

Joe: *All in all I loved my first PA house. I loved being there deep down. I probably did not show my appreciation properly. It was a fantastic place to be. My first impression, when I went there in (November 19XX), was a religious one ... that we were like the early Christians hiding in the catacombs. I really did not have an overwhelming religious experience until I went there. I really felt that we were adherents to some strange religion and were being persecuted.*

BS: By the psychiatrists ... who were the Romans?

Joe: *Yeah, not so much psychiatry but the state. I think the state keeping us in mental hospitals.*

BS: So overall, from your experience in [the PA houses], were they preferable to being in a mental hospital?

Joe: *Yes it was. The best hospital I was in had a dormitory which had about 40 beds. It was very much like being in the army or in prison, whereas in my first PA house you could be creative, you had your freedom. Although I was not locked up in the mental hospital, it was a very regimented lifestyle. The charge nurse would come in the morning at 7–7.30am and rattle a bunch of keys and bang them on the end of your metal bed and say 'c'mon gentlemen, time to get up'. Everything was regimented. A friend of mine used to work in the kitchen and he used to get a hot knife and cut a pat of butter into equal portions. You were allowed one bit of butter per day. It was ... I never did National Service because I was too young. It must have been something like that so we chose freedom, we chose freedom ...*

... I think if we had one thing in common it would have been one's belief and desire for freedom and we wanted to be free above everything else.

Joe described his despondency regarding modern times and the age of individualism, which may contribute as to why communal living such as the PA houses may not be popular anymore. Although Joe was not

unhappy living in his own flat and was insistent that he would never give it up, the idea of living again in a PA house still held a fond place in his heart.

Joe: *You know, everybody just wants what's good for themselves, the idea of communal living just seemed not to appeal anymore. So when you say about having only two houses left it does not surprise me. People think differently these days, they don't want to live communally.*

BS: What is your view/idea of a PA house from your experience? Do you think these things should still continue albeit on an improved level? If improvements should be made, what should they be? Or if not, is there a different way of doing things?

Joe: *Well I suppose what I am saying is, the PA should take a long good hard look at whether there is actually a market for it because I don't think there is in this day and age. I don't think it is what people want to do, what they expect out of life. If there is a market for it and if people are clamouring to live like that and the PA do it very well, then yes, but maybe people don't think like that anymore.*

BS: What do you think people think like these days?

Joe: *Well, I mentioned the 'me generation'; people say everybody is out for themselves and the common group is not discussed and Thatcher says there is no such thing as society, individuals rule (laughs). We just found at the end of my third stay in my third PA house that there were not enough people who wanted to live there anymore. My first PA house* [that Joe stayed in] *was revolutionary – the biggest jump in consciousness since the Civil War, but as I say, I think of it as the Wild West, a new frontier.*

BS: Troubled but striving for something.

Joe: *Yeah … it's adventurous, but also dangerous and I think you have to be fit and healthy and strong to go in for it. I am (XX) years old and I am not going to give up this* [his flat] *for anything (laughs).*

Testimony of experience

BS: So you wouldn't go to another PA house now?

Joe: *Well I could be tempted actually because I believe in the ideals and I have no real criticism with the PA. I don't think of them badly at all. I think they did a splendid job. I hope you found your training to be enlightening and useful to you.*

BS: Yes, I found it very useful ...

Joe: *Possibly because people in the PA don't have to put a concerted effort into running houses leads them to squabble amongst themselves. If they had more houses they might be more single minded in what they were doing ...*

... The whole cause is something I still do believe in. I don't think about it all that much, but it is nice to know ... 40 years on and it's still causing controversy and people are still questioning what it means to be mad and what it means to be sane and what it means to be free.

BS: Any last words, reflections, happy memories? ... Would you do it all again? Would you do things differently?

Joe: *I was an enfant terrible and at the end of the day infants have to grow up and I don't know whether my time in the houses was part of being childish and that the responsible adult thing to do was to have nothing to do with that ... I don't know ... it's taught me things I can't put into words ... I would do it again, I would do it again but, I am not sure whether there is much of an opportunity to do anything like that again. As you say it's very much the question of just two houses now ... I think for me it was part of growing up from a very immature boy into a more solidly based thinking person ... it was a second childhood because my first one was such a mess ... I needed a second one. I watched a TV programme about the Clouds rehab centre and a girl was talking about having been given a great opportunity and I thought ... very few people are given the opportunity to express themselves exactly as they want ... and I thought, hang on a minute ... I had that opportunity and it is a very rare precious thing that I have been given and she is right ... we live in a very regimented society and she said the ability to be just yourself which she experienced at the rehab centre. She pointed out very few people are granted that and I thought I was given that,*

I was granted that. I must count myself very, very fortunate to have been given such a wonderful opportunity and be careful not to waste it, which is why I am very pleased to have talked to you today. You know I want my experience to count for something, because very few people are given the opportunity I had and it just doesn't happen in most people's lives.

Chapter Nine

Rob

Rob is another ex-resident who found the PA community house-living experience very difficult, but, surprisingly, a very positive one. The idea of the paradox of struggle leading to certain resolutions of his problems became evident during our interview. His warmth, like Joe, in his descriptions about the PA and its house therapists, was very moving to hear.

Rob: *I think once I visited the PA I felt this was what I needed, rather than the (X)* [another organisation that offered communal living where Rob had stayed previously], *which was a bit more institutionalised. You had to go home at weekends so the fact that you could live at the PA all week had more appeal. And I liked the whole spirit of the house. People would sit there and have a go at you. There was something very real about it, something very raw. It felt like there was something really going on there and I really quite enjoyed that. The energy was very high; not like the previous place* [a therapeutic community] *I lived. There was not the same energy or focus on therapy there as there was in the PA.*

BS: What are your experiences in the house that were memorable?

Rob: *It's difficult, I am still in therapy and I was telling my therapist how difficult it is to actually give a coherent account of it all … because I feel differently about it at different times. In terms of being able to move on and my functioning, I feel it was very helpful. I have not had a breakdown since and I have held a job ever since. In that sense the therapy was very, very effective … But I found the group therapy* [the house meetings] *dysfunctional.*

Rob believed that the difficulty of living in the PA house was that as one was living with other people for a long time, blind spots started forming and it became difficult to see what was actually going on between people. However, paradoxically this was a helpful experience. Issues of coming to a point to 'make up one's own mind' became evident.

BS: If I understand you right, because you are with the same people for a long time, blind spots start forming?

Rob: *I think so. I don't think you necessarily respond in a mature way because you find yourself thinking, oh it's just that particular person, and of course there is that personal level. Some people are a fucking pain in the arse and you live with them year in, year out and you hear their problems a thousand times. You hear them taking out their negative projections on you a thousand times and you end up just hating them. Living in the house was a fucking nightmare. It was also very powerful and helpful. I wish I could sit here and give you a tidy response. In some way I miss the rawness of it and the real struggle to be honest* [the effort of being honest]. *When I had your email I kind of got excited because I had not had any contact with the PA for about two years. It is, the experience of the houses, is something that I have not experienced outside the houses. It was tremendously rich and it was a mixture of total fucking boredom, growth, and transformation all mixed up together. But you get sick of people who have not done the washing up, even though probably everyone has not done a bit of it. Everybody is looking for a bogeyman. You go on holiday for a week and everyone decides to wash up because they want to blame you. You come back and find you are being blamed for the washing up because everyone has colluded to do the washing up while you have been on holiday. I think I stayed in the house too long although I think I did a lot of work in the house in the last year. That was very powerful. Who is in the house really affects the amount of work you do and how engaged you are. That really got me moving and woke me up ... in a way that I had not realised to the other residents. But I did feel that six years was too long and I did not think I was that ill that I had to stay there for six years.*

The ethos of the PA was one reason why Rob was satisfied with his stay in a PA house. He was sympathetic to the critical and questioning

stance taken by the PA and its therapists to psychiatry and psychiatric medication.

BS: You have probably heard about the historical legacy of the PA: Laing etc., alternative ways of living, no medication, anti-psychiatry, that sort of thing. What were the views on medication in the house?

Rob: *Well, I was very convinced by the therapists' views on it, but the actual therapists themselves stopped short of saying to people that they should not take their medication. They were very, very careful about how they worded it. They would support people coming off medication. They would raise questions about it. But they did it very delicately. I very much bought into the idea of no medication. I did not want to have medication and when I went to the PA, I just thought, what a breath of fresh air, you know, inspiring. I was totally convinced by it, but then again I was not that ill, so ...*

BS: Obviously a lot of people come to the house with a label; e.g., depression. Are these labels important in the house?

Rob: *No, quite the opposite. They sort of brushed them away and again personally I found that very, very helpful.*

The difficulty of living in the house, the paradox of this difficulty, and the suffering attached to this was again highlighted during our conversation.

BS: In terms of structure ... you had the group meetings, the living experience ... from when you went in until you left, what do you think were the helpful things that you felt you got out of living in the house?

Rob: *I became much more aware that other people existed. I was much more able to think about myself in relation to other people rather than being stuck in my own world. I think I matured quite a bit. I started to take more responsibility for my reactions to things. I had quite deep-rooted difficulties which moved forward a lot in the house and as a distinct result of getting involved with people having had tremendous difficulties. Very, very intense, awful ... that all changed* [it improved for Rob in the house].

BS: So do you think there was much community spirit there?

Rob: *No, it was a totally loveless place. In terms of the residents there was no love really but I think there was a lot of unloved people there which contributed to no love being shown or offered … that's just where they were you know and I would not idealise the house at all. It was a fucking nightmare to live in. There was more of a spirit, more of an understanding of it at the beginning; it was just residents in the house and there was the idea that you got into some really heavy shit with people and afterwards you would forgive each other and you would use each other to work, to do the work and it gets quite difficult. But the later people came in and they just did not want to do that. There was a desire to maintain equilibrium. There was a culture where before the Monday evening meeting we would have a meal and the Monday evening meeting was like the flash point of the week. That's when everyone would blow up. And this was kind of like a collusion to break the tension; let's make everything OK. So I did not like the group I was in at all. But that was partly because the dominant male in the house absolutely hated me and wanted to kill me – so probably now if I was pushed I would be more aware of the dynamics and be a lot more thoughtful about, 'well maybe I am in this position of scapegoat because the dominant male is out to get me and I am being sidelined' … I would be more political about it now.*

BS: Its sounds quite a journey?

Rob: *It was a fucking nightmare to live in that house, a fucking nightmare. The weird thing is I kind of miss it. I miss the intensity of it. It was a bit like living in the 1960s. The therapists were all kind of from the late 60s and they like broke every fucking rule in the book and I think they were quite brilliant, quite brilliant and it was what I liked about the houses … is that they* [the house therapists] *would take risks and they would go off … they wouldn't just cover their own backs, they would take risks and break the rules.*

The topic of the unorthodox way of working by the PA therapists was something that Rob felt was important about the way the PA communities were run.

Rob: *A therapist would come ... a therapist might talk about their drug taking. So that's what was so wonderful about it ... you really felt that they were trying to give you what you needed, rather than ... and actually I didn't take drugs in the house at all, but a few years ago I took a load of magic mushrooms ... and it was incredibly useful and therapeutic. I remember one of the therapists coming to a meeting and telling us how the previous evening he had taken magic mushrooms on Hampstead Heath. I remember being quite shocked by this but when I tried them* [magic mushrooms] *myself I just thought they were tremendously therapeutic, but there was a period during the trip where I was incredibly ill. It was a bit like being in the 1960s living in the house.*

Although Rob found the therapists extremely helpful, he found the 'psychoanalytic framework' that the house therapists used difficult to deal with. But strangely this struggle again led Rob to come to his own mind, eventually leave, and seek other means of help; the struggle (or accepting one was in it) led him like the fly to get out of the bottle.

Rob: *I think towards the end I felt a bit manipulated by the type of therapy they used ... they would be using you to get at somebody's projections. You really felt they were playing snooker with people in the house and that was fine for a few years because you don't notice them doing it. But after about five to six years you begin to feel a bit manipulated and one of my main issues was that I found my mother to be very evasive. So I think why the therapy was a failure is because there was something very deep in me that could not accept being pushed around and forced into particular different responses and stuff. They reminded me of my mother being very evasive and I am in a different kind of therapy now which is not like that.*

BS: When you mean your therapy failed, do you mean your individual therapy or the house?

Rob: *The group therapy, the house meetings. I started to withdraw from the therapy I think and I think I was being pushed into different positions and I was being manipulated slightly. The aim of the therapists was to resolve issues between residents and I felt sometimes I was being manipulated and I felt sometimes my interests were being sacrificed because they focused on something else. I remember someone having a go at me and I remember feeling quite separate from what they were into. And the therapists pushed me into it and I actually felt it was nothing to do with me. It may partly have had something to do with me but I felt very clearly that this chap was just going off on one. I felt like I was being pulled into other people's places and madness sometimes because that person needed me or someone else to engage with them.*

BS: So back to the last question ... what were the things you felt you did not get from the house?

Rob: *I didn't feel ... able to make ... I felt less able to make friends after I left. I don't know whether that was because I was going more deeply into stuff ... you know ... that I was becoming more grounded or real as a result of the experience in the house ... I felt very much scapegoated and isolated. So that side of it was not very helpful ... I know in some ways I felt I was being hit with a sledgehammer and it did resolve some very deep issues which caused my breakdown in the first place ... So I don't know if I left the house with things just partially resolved or whether I was quite damaged with this experience ... I think also, I think the working world ... I was quite disrespectful of it. I thought by being in the house ... I think they were very good at managing our self-esteem given the fact that we had mental health problems and were unemployed. They were very good at making us feel that we were very meaningful and very rich and quite privileged ... something that most people never have a chance to go through. But I also came away with looking down on the working world.*

The lack of a formalised structure and the PA house therapists' use of a psychoanalytic-type frame may have led to much anger and confusion for Rob, but it also seems that it may have been helpful. This appears paradoxical. He talked later about the house therapists, and the paradox of suffering leading to salvation again shone from a quite implicit place.

BS: Sounds like there was a real blurring that the roles were not that well defined?

Rob: *I felt that the therapists had very clear boundaries, but they were not formalised. They were not at a guidebook level; legalistic boundaries. They were intuitive boundaries and they were much more powerful because of that. You did not feel that there was an us and them in the way that you might find elsewhere.*

… It was really weird. They wanted you to have all your energy in the house and be involved with these people who you might not be necessarily interested in but you were supposed to invest as much of your energy in the house as possible.

BS: So you were not encouraged to even go and get voluntary work?

Rob: *No I wasn't encouraged. They would not stop you but … The house therapist just was not interested in doing voluntary work at all. I did not feel encouraged in that at all.*

BS: What did they expect you to do all day? Just hang around the house?

Rob: *There was no sense of rush – which was great when you started so you could relax and settle into the house. I think they would have been quite happy for you to have been there for ten years. It wasn't necessary for some people. It wasn't necessary for me; I needed to be there about four years. It just wasn't necessary.*

BS: Any last thoughts or reflections about your stay in the community?

Rob: *I feel so incredibly grateful. I feel I was able to function and move on and you know, not be a mental case despite the fact I still have ongoing problems but I am still in therapy but they sort of went to an effort. They* [the PA house therapists] *didn't worry too much about following some stupid guidebook to cover their own backs. You really felt they were doing what they could to help you. It was a very strange experience and I will always be grateful.* [Rob at this point was very tearful, in a joyful way.]

Chapter Ten

Rose

Rose is an ex-psychiatric hospital patient who found her way to the PA.

Rose: *In the hospital in (a town) I saw an alternative psychologist. I can't remember why or how. He thought I shouldn't be in the place that I was. It certainly was furthering me away from the person I felt that I should be. I felt I was being treated sadistically and this precipitated panic breakdown. So being in that hospital furthered me from myself, not being in touch with who I am and that furthered me from myself. I heard about a place called the PA and I ran away from that hospital because I thought if I stayed there I would have been there until I was an old lady. The things that were happening there were furthering me into panic; not being treated like a human being, other people around me were complete and utter vegetables and suffering from tardive dyskinsia from the effects of antipsychotic drugs. I only ever had Valium because of panic attacks. Anyway, I left the place and I changed my name to my original name which is (XX) and I never went back to (that hospital) again. I hitched a lift, I didn't have any money, I didn't have any other clothes other than the clothes I was in and I left the past behind. Not quite as simple as that and I was only 26 at the time ...*

After getting to London in quite a distressed state she found the PA but it was not the experience or set-up she had hoped for.

Rose: *... Anyway to cut a long story short I stayed with somebody I sort of knew and she paid for me to go and see (a PA therapist) which was in (a part of London). One of the members of the house was there (X). (The PA therapist) asked me if I would like to go into a place called (the PA house). I didn't know, I* *was numb in myself and I didn't know what to say. They* [the PA therapist and my friend] *wanted me to make up my mind because (X)* [a fellow resident who was in the building and was getting ready to drive back to the PA house] *couldn't be very long and he could go back with me. I said I would. I had to make some decision in my life and I didn't know and I didn't know what to do. I could have stayed where I was for a while but the lady I was staying with couldn't. It's a long story; I won't go into it ...*

... It became apparent when I got there ... there were six people who had been there already and they really didn't want a seventh person. But the PA people like (PA therapist 1, PA therapist 2) and maybe (PA therapist 3) ... I didn't speak to anybody ... it really was meant for people who had been in hospital and were suffering from some kind of breakdown or distress, of which I had and did. So they didn't want anybody there with any real problems. I mean the people that were there arguing amongst each other. There was a house divided between (several people). So I went to a house that was already divided. It was like being in family having dreadful rows. It was a very traumatic place to be in, especially having gone there in complete trust thinking it would be a place of security; it was a very, very scary place to be and there was not enough security to be had outwardly from anyone in there. The only security net I had was that at least I had a nook of my own and that was something. But there were a lot of strong characters in there that were vehemently against anyone else being there. So I was vulnerable and it was very difficult to survive in a place like that. I was attacked by someone. But there was no one I was able to talk to and express what was going on. It was worse than staying in a ... it was worse than the worst of dysfunctional families and I was there for three-and-a-half years ... it was the most anarchistic place. Anybody could do anything to anybody and get away with anything. It was certainly a very frightening place to be. It didn't do my panic attacks, my nervous anxiety, any good whatsoever.

Rose found the argumentative environment very stressful but tried (in vain it seems) to help create peace.

Rose: *I always tried to be peacemaker throughout my life and maintain my own integrity. It was nice to be needed ...* [Rose then went on to describe how a fellow ex-resident asked her to look after her children] ... *But the building was in total disarray and there were so many rows and I was not a part of any of it. I would always stay away. In fact I stayed in my room for a year or more, never venturing out because of all the rows, turmoil and noise. So it was safer to stay in my bedroom and then I would only go downstairs when nobody was around and then help myself to food. But that would concur with 'why don't you like us?' attitude* [questions from other residents of the house about Rose's seclusion in her room] ... *and I couldn't really say* [to the other residents why she secluded herself] *as I have never been a confrontational person. It was no good telling other people why. I wanted to stay away from it all and didn't want to be stuck in the situation of not seeing the woods from the trees, as they were. Yes it was very difficult not to get immersed in somebody's mess in the house ...*

Rose did not find the group therapeutic support effective for herself. It seemed she would have liked to have more of a one-to-one therapeutic experience but this was not on offer.

Rose: *He was very cerebral* [the house therapist]. *He never really ... he had to be I suppose as they were so many people around him. I never felt that he was really listening to you. I had one occasion to be with (the house therapist) alone. I felt then that he really had understood me. He gave me some sound advice. I wish I had been able to talk with him about things on my own. I am sure that would have been a lot better than the group experience. In the group experience I found myself disappearing more and more and staring out the window or looking at flowers or doing something to distract myself from the stress of the arguing. So I didn't find the group situation and meetings very helpful and neither did anybody else. There would be full-scale rows happening between everybody and I would just stare out the window and just block off mentally as I always do really when things get too much. I didn't join in with any of it. (The house therapist) used to come round to me and say, 'What do you think?' I can't remember if I said anything.*

BS: You were there for three-and-a-half years. Were you ever encouraged to get into individual psychotherapy?

Rose: *There wasn't anything like that. You've got to be joking. If a human being could survive living there* [in the PA house], *one could survive living anywhere. I certainly learned a lot about human nature and the bad side of human nature. Nobody was on medication except me I think. I was on lorazepam* [a psychiatric drug] *because my nerves were so bad.*

Towards the end of the interview, Rose brought up the interesting point of spirituality and how she had seen the ethos of the PA, which was not fulfilled in how she experienced the house.

Rose: *It's interesting … I heard a story at the PA – 'Behold I have set before you an open door and no man shall shut it'* [a quote from one of the PA advertising leaflets, originally from The New Testament, Book of Revelation, 3:8]. *I wish there had been more of a philosophy based on spiritual disciplines in the house. I wish there had been* [more of a spiritual dimension in the PA house] *… you know you* [the author, before our interview began] *talked about Buddhism … I wish there had been more Buddhism or Christian people who believed in spiritual matters, the love of God and shown that to one another. But people didn't want to know about spiritual matters either. I think it's a shame that it* [the house] *didn't work out.*

BS: I see what you mean … the PA espouses a kind of Christian/Buddhist ethics, but it didn't seem to be there in the community from your perspective.

Rose: *No, no … but even in the churches it is missing in some that I have experienced. We each have got to find our own way, our own path in our lives so at least there wasn't anyone there that was going to be badgered into anything. But I think it went too far the other way really. It could have been a middle ground. But there wasn't. So from my point of view there was none of the help that you can get today. But there was none whatsoever. Nuff said!*

Chapter Eleven

Julia

In the PA communities during the 60s and 70s (and on one rare occasion in recent history)[1] it was possible for residents to live-in with their children. Julia is one example where she came to live in a PA house when her mother moved in. There were also other children living there with their parents. Julia's account is important in demystifying the stigma (or even questioning the so-called concept) of mental illness and the scaremongering of the so-called risks and dangers of living in a house with people in varying states of mental distress.

Julia: *My experience of living there was mainly positive. There were several other children to play with and I loved all the animals. Two of the other children also had ponies so I learned to milk goats and ride ponies … Having come from a council estate in a large city with no pets, this was my first real experience of the countryside. I loved being around so much greenery, trees, flowers, blackberry picking, digging up potatoes, and picking fruit and 'veg' from the garden … It felt pretty safe most of the time. I think most of the adults kept an eye out for us kids. We were allowed quite a lot of freedom to roam around; pretty feral really, but there was always someone to keep an eye on us.*

The conversation then picked up on the idea that a PA community where parents in varying degrees of mental distress and their children come to stay may be beneficial for all parties owing to the communal support on offer.

Julia: *I think this helped Mum a lot with her stress levels* [that there was always someone to keep an eye on her kids]. *The adults included us quite a lot with everyday stuff like cooking, making cheese. They were mostly interested in us, showed us anything we took an interest in, woodwork, for example. I think they tried to help each other and be supportive mostly, although there were some who kept themselves apart because they were selfish or just lost in their own head or possibly to avoid conflict. I remember some of the men building and installing a shower downstairs and tiling it; there was a manly can-do attitude, let's have a go, which was positive.*

Obviously, like most 'normal' households in the world, the living environment is not a utopia. Julia's comments on what she found difficult and helpful from living in a PA house could be applicable to a conventional family set-up.

BS: What did you find difficult about living in a PA community house, and what was positive and helpful?

Julia: [What she found positive] *The communal atmosphere, other children, lots of outdoor space, freedom, healthy food and fresh air …* [And unhelpful or difficult] *Not understanding adult relationships, occasional arguments between adults were scary, I didn't understand them. No one sat us down and explained stuff to us … the attitudes outside the house … kids treated us differently* [children who lived in the community outside the PA house]. *My sister was a teenager and I think it was particularly hard for her. Not having much money, not having a lot of interaction with the outside community …*

Julia offered her ideas of what could have been improved about the community she lived in.

Julia: *I think that there should have been more one-to-one therapy for the adults. I think that the fact that there were children there should have been thought about more carefully, maybe monitored. I think I would have benefited from some therapy too. My parents divorced while I was there which was very upsetting and confusing for me. My sister was very distressed at that time also; no one really picked up on our emotional difficulties. Having had problems with depression as a teen and adult, it could have been helpful and preventative for me and other children to have an assessment of our emotional needs, and a check-up.*

BS: Would you recommend the experience of living in the house for people suffering from mental distress and if so why?

Julia: *I would with perhaps a bit more structure and monitoring in place ... when it worked it was great.*

BS: Is it any better or worse [the PA houses] than the alternatives? If so why?

Julia: *From what I have seen of mental health services as an adult personally, and professionally* [in her job within the mental health field] *there was a family and community atmosphere that wasn't clinical; a more natural way to help people heal. People were encouraged to get on and do things for themselves, make stuff, fix things, grow their own food. I've seen this in a watered-down version on psychiatric wards with OT* [occupational therapy] *sessions, they are more like add-ons; patients don't cook their own dinner, they have cooking lessons or sessions. They don't build stuff for the ward or their home; they make a piece of arts and crafts that is expressive, but separate from real life. There needs to be a crossover, some kind of middle ground I think, to keep people attached to reality.*

Julia then discussed why a PA community like she stayed in as a child may not be able to exist.

Julia: *I think that the PA house I stayed in was of its time ... nowadays people are more afraid, authorities are scared of being sued if things go wrong and are only interested in providing the bare minimum at the least cost. There seems to be no quality of care. 'Community care'[2] just doesn't seem to work; there are a lot of isolated people out there suffering from mental health difficulties.*

Endnotes
1. A resident gave birth to a baby in the Shirland Road community, London. This community closed in 2005 because of funding pressures.
2. This is a reference to the government's policy, 'Care in the Community', and one of the organisations who run it, Supporting People.

Chapter Twelve

Simon

Simon is an ex-resident who seems to represent the kind of person who was not suited to PA community houses. There were some reasons that he voiced as to why this was the case along with some of the difficulties that he experienced in trying to integrate and find his voice in the house. Simon now lives in his own flat. He does not work and is not in receipt of any psychiatric or psychological care but is considering getting some further help.

Simon: *I have had therapy in the past and I found it very helpful but I still had some hang-ups, paranoia and confusion. I could not understand why and so I went into the PA house to help with this and my social communication problems, to find out about my psychological blocks and if anything could be done to remove them. But that never happened in the ten months I was there. One reason this might have been is that one of the residents seemed to say more than anyone else. I did speak a few times and one of those times it seemed like she was telling me off because of what I said. I thought I was being insightful. So this made me modest about speaking in the house meetings.*

BS: Are you saying that you found the meetings difficult?

Simon: *Yes. The last few months I was in the house I started to see this therapist called (XX) at (an organisation). He was a teacher of psychology theory or something. When I was silent he kind of forced me to speak and it seemed to work and we started communicating and understanding each other. So I was thinking the PA should maybe have a rule for people before they move into the house; everybody should have a ten- to fifteen-minute slot to say something and nobody interrupts no matter what thoughts and feelings they may have. That might be helpful to the therapy ... I don't know... it could be.*

BS: That's interesting. So you feel that some people dominated house meetings. Was this problem not addressed by the house therapists?

Simon: *Yes.*

But there were aspects of Simon's stay that were of a positive nature.

Simon: *I started to like the people there immediately, but as I said, the house never solved this problem I had with communication. But being there did help me with my paranoia about not being liked or being disrespected ... I realised that I was liked and respected by the other residents to some degree.*

BS: So do you think it helped you with some aspects of your self-esteem?

Simon: *Self-esteem ... yes.*

Simon's reasons for leaving the PA house after a relatively short stay were a mixture of 'therapeutic preferences' and external influences.

BS: So why did you leave the house?

Simon: *Well, um ... I started to become interested in a lot of other stuff. I got into NLP* [neuro-linguistic programming, a type of psychotherapy] *and got books out on it. I made my mind up that I had to get over my problems myself because my father kept phoning up and said, 'Oh you had better watch out, you are going to become homeless, they are barrack room boys those people at the PA.'*

BS: What are barrack room boys?

Simon: *It's some kind of insult, I don't know.*

BS: I've never heard that one before. So you say that your dad was not happy about where you were? He thought that the PA people were a bit whacky?

Simon: *Yes.*

BS: So you thought you could do it by yourself and you thought you could just move out? But you were not told to leave?

Simon: *Yes ... you see I was not sleeping properly, concentrating properly, I was confused. I had a problem with my blood, I thought it was. I was worrying too much and drinking in the evenings. Then I found out what was wrong and the doctor gave me medication for high blood pressure or something. So I am not totally better now but I am a lot better now. I left under a cloud of confusion; I threatened another resident and said I would hit him. I left that same night, but I later apologised to him.*

BS: So you left under a cloud of bad blood between this person and yourself.

Simon: *Yes.*

Although Simon experienced great difficulties with the 'working' of the house, his communication problems, and therapeutic preferences that were not met, he did find his stay of some help, but revealed that his difficulty in 'getting into' the PA house may have been due to his expectation that therapists should have all the answers.

BS: You have already said that you found the house meetings difficult. What else did you find difficult?

Simon: *I struggled with my cooking skills, but another resident used to help me sometimes. My communication problem was difficult to deal with.*

BS: On the flip side what did you find helpful about living in the house?

Simon: *My self-esteem went up, the house helped that.*

BS: Do you think there was any particular reason why the house did this? What do you think it was?

Simon: *Living with other people. Not being frightened of having problems, not being frightened of* [being] *judged as being psychological. So living with other people helped me. I tried my best to support and understand them, they did their best to support and understand me.*

BS: How did you feel the house therapists treated you and how did you feel if it was compared to different types of 'treatment' you have had experience of?

Simon: *Well when I once saw a trainee psychotherapist she seemed to know a lot about me before I even told her much about me from what I explained about what my parents were like. And I never found that from the therapists in the house. Or maybe because I never spoke much in the house meetings. That's the only difference that I can think of. They never had as much insight into me as I would have liked.*

BS: The house therapists, you thought they should have had more insight into you?

Simon: *Yes. They see things and interpret things how they see and interpret the world as I see things and interpret things how I see the world. Sometimes misunderstandings happen.*

Simon did express some regrets that may have contributed to the house therapists not having enough insight into him as he had hoped, but again reiterated that it seemed he wanted didactic therapeutic support.

Simon: *I just wished that I had spoken a lot more. I just wish that the house therapists had had more insight into me and said things like my old psychotherapist like … unconscious stuff to do with my family. My old psychotherapist told me that my parents' strange behaviour was due to their childhood. I am convinced if they* [the house therapists] *had had more insight into me they would have been able to help me.*

Having ascertained that the ethos and/or working of the PA house was not entirely to his liking, I enquired as to what he thought the ethos of way of working was in a PA house and what he would change, if anything.

BS: What did you feel the philosophy of the PA was? Can you describe what you felt the PA was all about, their ethos?

Simon: *No I don't understand why people … well I don't know if it is necessary for people in the house for their self-esteem or mental health. All I know is that people with mental health problems or psychological problems or people that are stuck need a lot more help in this country. There is more to our problems than meets the eye or how we happen to be. Those of us who have this insight are not getting the right sort of help that we need. At least the PA is at least doing something. I don't know if it's the right thing or not but at least it's doing something.*

BS: So you felt that the PA was trying to do something that was quite important then?

Simon: *Yes.*

BS: Apart from what you have already said, are there any recommendations you could give the PA? How would you change things, if you could go back, what would you change?

Simon: *Maybe a combination of psychotherapy and CBT* [is needed in the PA houses] *so people can change their negative and irrational beliefs. Because otherwise you have got to work it out for yourself. Like my old therapist said to me, 'How can I conquer this?', I mean even if you accept it, so I did. How can I work it out, how can I think differently?*

BS: So a different type of therapy rather than what the PA offers, because it might not suit everyone I suppose?

Simon: *Yes.*

Chapter Thirteen

Sally

A common story I heard from the people I interviewed was that the period just prior to entering a PA house was a time where the prospective resident had felt near rock bottom and that a big change in their lives was needed. It felt to me that for many it was the cry of the last chance. This is Sally's story.

Sally: *Just before I was looking at (PA house) I was in a crisis. I had reached a point where I wanted to do something quite ... I needed to make a big change ... I knew I wanted to live with other people ... but knew it needed to be a supportive environment ... I had been living on my own and so I was very isolated and then I was living with a woman who took me in out of kindness of her heart really. I had been working part time for over a year ... but then I just completely broke down, and I stopped working. I was just in a bit of a mess really. I was just looking for a fresh start. But that was ... I had had a long, long history of mental health issues since I was a child.*

Sally found the transition from moving into the PA house quite difficult. It was by no means an easy option despite her desperate feelings.

Sally: *I found it very hard to use them* [the house meetings] *to begin with. I was terrified and I would often just sit and I didn't feel able to participate and I would often go in with my little piece of paper with things written down that I wanted to say but I didn't manage to say. I was kind of wanting people to help me to sort of ... you know ... get into the meetings. But that was rarely the case and certainly the therapists didn't make any effort. People actually started complaining that I didn't speak in the meetings and it was not a deliberate thing.*

I just found it really, really intense and I don't know, as time went on ... it seemed like it was just the same old thing being said over and over again by people ... there are a lot of issues around anger ... and I found that quite difficult.

BS: What was the anger about?

Sally: *People were feeling angry towards their family, the way their parents brought them up ... their parents having created their difficulties that they had now and people would ... sometimes people would encourage me to ... they felt I should be dwelling more on my upbringing and how that impacted. But I was kind of quite reluctant I suppose. But, because ... you know I had had therapy for years and years ... I kind of had really gone over all this stuff so much and I kind of felt like I had put a lot of it to rest and people were wanting me to dig it all up again and I found that quite hard.*

BS: What were the therapists' ideas on this about dragging up the family?

Sally: *They seemed to encourage me as well, definitely, and they kind of ... I really felt kind of that people told me that I was kind of avoiding stuff, avoiding the real issues and how like ... how could I be positive about anything when such bad things had happened to me ... you know ... because I still had issues and stuff ... I really found it hard that there was not encouragement in looking forward, to achieving things at the time and things outside the house. I did voluntary work and things and I didn't think it went down all that well ... and I was like well, surely this is kind of a very positive step.*

BS: It didn't go down well with the therapists or the residents?

Sally: *Both really ... they felt I should be putting all my time and effort into the house. And for me that just wasn't a valid life. Everything being about therapy and the house, you could have too much therapy.*

This theme of getting stuck in to the routine of the house (i.e., the meetings and ordinary daily living) and the difficulty of doing so were reflected later in the interview.

Sally: *There were forever arguments about the washing up and cleaning rotas and watering the garden etc. So it was like all those things could never be straightforward. They were all interpreted, they were all made into those complicated things and sometimes that got too much for me. I mean, why can't cleaning the house just be cleaning the house? ... because it was quite ... some people didn't care about cleaning while for others it was very important.*

Sally explained that much of the ordinary living in the house involved the running of the house as any other household would have to, and that this could become complicated as it involved negotiation between residents.

BS: What about house maintenance and decoration? How was this carried out?

Sally: *Well we kind of ... it was left up to us. We found people to come in and do the work and then we gave the invoices to (the house therapists). But we had to do all the research and then order it and everything and get them to pay for it. But again it seemed like it was left down to a few people in the house. A lot of people didn't even care if we had a fridge or not. To me that was something really important so I got on and did it.*

BS: So you had to basically run the houses yourself really.

Sally: *Yeah, we did really.*

BS: It sounds like you had a lot of responsibility?

Sally: *Yeah ... and that was just the cause of endless rows and everything in the meetings. Somebody* [another resident] *again didn't want anything to do with it* [residents were given some money by the PA to buy an item of furniture]. *It literally became such a complicated thing ... the therapists were not going to get involved with the practical side of it at all and in some ways it was nice to do what we wanted with the money but it was complicated.*

B: A lot of negotiation?

Testimony of experience

Sally: *Yeah ...*

Although the PA espouses the philosophy and ethos of community, unfortunately, Sally was disappointed with her experience of the lack of community spirit in the house.

Sally: *One of the things about the PA was that there were the meetings ... but I wished there had been more creative things, more sense of community and things to encourage that. The only thing we tried was to have a meal together. I think on a Sunday, but for a long time there was no meal at all. Maybe some people would come, some wouldn't, and there was the whole thing about who was going to cook. Again it became a really complicated affair that was not going to be enjoyed. And to me that felt such a shame.*

Whilst living in the house, Sally, during her personal psychotherapy, also visited a psychiatrist every once in a while. She described her experience of psychiatry in the interview. One must bear in mind that psychiatric diagnosis does not play a big part in the ethos of the PA. From a phenomenological standpoint what presents itself (e.g., a person's distress and what is going on for them) is how (it seems) the house therapists deal with things.

BS: Did he [the psychiatrist] provide much input?

Sally: *Not really ... he dealt with my medication ... I discovered after a few months of moving to London that I had been diagnosed with (a psychiatric disorder) ... I was never told this before. Apparently this was written in my notes by my psychiatrist without anybody telling me anything. I was very shocked they would do that. I remember I went back to a meeting and they told me I have (a psychiatric disorder),* [and that] *it was written in my notes and the house therapists were very nonplussed about it really ... and I was like ... do I have this? ... do I have it? ... and somehow it was important that I had been given this label.*

Sally found the 'groundlessness' of not having her psychiatric diagnosis confirmed by the house therapists quite alarming. In other words it seemed she was left to work it out for herself. This led to the helpfulness

of the paradox of struggling and coming to 'one's own mind' about certain things.

BS: What did you find helpful about living in the house?

Sally: *It was really learning to live with other people .. it was really, really good ... it was hard but ... just for me, learning about social interaction ... it was quite important and in the end I kind of felt like to me it was good for me to stop and see that actually these meetings didn't help me or at least they don't help me anymore and I actually don't agree with this you know ... the way that the therapists were working and for me to actually stand up and say this isn't what I want ... I want to move on was really important for me ... to make that decision ... but I have very mixed feelings about the whole experience really but I don't totally regret it. Coming to London gave me that fresh start I needed and for me getting the space from where I grew up and my family and everything was really good. And trying to learn how to speak during the meetings, what I felt about things. But what I think really benefited me more was from what other residents in the house said, more than what the therapists said.*

This difficulty of making up one's own mind was further illuminated later on during the interview when finding out what Sally found unhelpful about her stay in the house.

BS: So what was unhelpful about the experience of living in the house?

Sally: *Lack of encouragement to do things. You know in terms of people wanting to move on getting voluntary work or even a paid job, of making friends and relationships outside the house, to take you out more. I mean those things should be encouraged more because of the lack of a sense of community in the house and the lack of all those other things, apart from the meetings you need to look outside for those things also.*

BS: Interesting ... so you became frustrated with this state of affairs and you felt you had to make your own mind up and just go for it despite what others thought?

Sally: *Yeah ... yeah ... but in some ways for me that was quite good ... it gave me more confidence ... to think actually this is what I want to do ... and you know I am actually going to do it ... despite the fact that you* [the house therapists] *don't agree ... I was terrified to say that* [to the house therapists] *but I did ... and you know I do feel that I absolutely made the right decision to go there at the time* [the PA house] *and make the* [correct] *decision to leave when I did.*

BS: Sounds like it's a bit of a paradox really?

Sally: *It is really ... because I don't want to totally say I don't like the house,* [that] *it didn't do me any good or anything, because it was not like that. I don't want to come over as if it was all negative, but for me there were a lot of negative things but not everything.*

In the course of the interview Sally told me that for some people a PA house might not be appropriate but that for others it would be. I then proceeded to ask her what she thought about the alternatives that exist.

Sally: *I have been in supported housing. It was time limited for a year and it was OK, but obviously there is none of the therapeutic element in that. It was more about how you were getting on with living independently ... I mean I did have a key worker, we did talk a little bit about how my health was and what other support I was getting. There was no sort of ... you were not really encouraged to be in therapy or anything especially ... it just so happened that I was. It was OK but it wasn't ... I think there were five or six flats but I didn't ... you really didn't get to know the other people or anything really. It wasn't bad but it was very, very, very different from the PA house. I mean I think it's got to be a lot better than hospital.*

BS: Have you had an experience of hospital?

Sally: *I have, quite a few years ago. But I think, when I was at (the PA house) one resident, she became very unwell. The therapists really didn't want her to go into hospital unless it was absolutely necessary, but that kind of put a huge weight on us ... the other residents. We were literally looking after her ... we had to lock* the doors because she would run outside. She was completely out of it. In the end she had to go into hospital ... we just couldn't look after her. But I have not been in a hospital in London. When we visited her in the hospital it just seemed horrible, really horrible.*

BS: In what way was it horrible?

Sally: *Well, it just seemed so depressing; you didn't have your own room or anything and the person we were going to see was just so highly medicated. And that just seemed so sad really. The whole place just seemed so depressing, really negative.*

Like other people I interviewed, Sally felt that she wanted more one-to-one time with the house therapists and that there was a lack of other activities, but there was too much focus on therapy – the group/house meetings.

Sally: *I don't think so ... the therapists were there for the meetings ... there was no real opportunity ... we were each allocated one of the therapists ... we would meet with them not very often ... literally every few months and it was literally to fill out forms ... it was more for paper work I think. Sometimes I wished there had been more opportunity for one-to-one with them ... especially when I was really struggling to say things in the meetings. It would have been nice to speak to one of the therapists ... it might have been helpful.*

BS: You also mentioned right at the start that other than the house meetings there were no other activities going on. Is that another thing you think they could improve on?

Sally: *Yeah I think so. More activities where people could enjoy themselves a bit ... people didn't believe me when I said I enjoyed things, especially like creative things. It was so frustrating ... they were like how could you possibly enjoy anything when you have got these problems, this background ... personally I do believe you can separate yourself a bit from your mental health stuff.*

BS: It sounds like there was a kind of obsession of dwelling in mental health stuff?

Sally: *I think when I was in the house it got stuck ... I felt when I was there it was going round in circles, a bit stale ... I suppose it really does depend who is there, how long they have been there, and who the therapists are.*

Chapter Fourteen

Thomas

Thomas is another ex-resident who found and came to the PA via the influence of R.D. Laing, from his writing and public fame.

Thomas: *So, first, I went to hear a lecture by R.D. Laing in (a library) in (October 19XX) and he was speaking about the PA houses, the philosophy behind them and the strategies that they had with this approach and in the break I went up to him and introduced myself and asked if I could give him a call. I told him I was a student from (a country). I also asked him about Wittgenstein because my tutor at university was very enthusiastic about him and didn't know Laing was still alive. Ronnie [Laing] was still alive (laughs) after his experience in Sri Lanka. So he [Laing] said give me a call and I did eventually and I asked if I could go into the house. He said yes but I would have to come and see him first, which I did. He gave me some of his time and we had a chat in his office and he said I would have to formally apply* [in writing]. *So I did. So I did apply and I was given two interviews ... I enjoyed living and working in (another community)* [that Thomas had lived in previously] *... I felt the PA houses were probably more open and congenial to some people's way of living, after having been influenced by the story of Mary Barnes*[1] *and the fact that I had seen the film about the Archway community where Leon Redler was and other people ... Asylum*[2] *that was the film ... so that was my motivation to go into the houses.*

Although the ethos of the PA houses in Thomas's time was one where there was supposedly no hierarchy, the emergence of a hierarchy inevitably leaked through. The idea of entering into a fairly chaotic household came to the fore in Thomas's description of the house, but

also of finding one's own rhythm – the ethos of the PA houses in some way – autorhythmia. Furthermore, the idea of struggle to find one's own autorhythmia became clear.

Thomas: *So one could only enter as a patient, well in the house nobody was called a patient, but someone who is looking for therapeutic community … It was a kind of positive identification and yet I also had to get adjusted to the habits. In the house there was also a hierarchy of who had been living there the longest, who was most mad. I did not know that in the beginning, but later I clearly sussed this out. This is a hierarchy of pain and luckily we had a secretary at the community who collected rent and who turned up once a week so we could discuss small things with her* [e.g., maintenance]. *But I also felt to be a bit of an outsider. I was a foreigner although there were other non-British there too. So I started to see the sociology of the houses.*

[Thomas then described how the house therapists tried to help a very withdrawn resident.] *She reminded me of somebody being a star patient. I found this very anarchic and very unjust, very unjust. I was just starting to work things out in there, what's right, what's just, what's the ethics of living a good life, the day-to-day life as you asked, cleaning the house, being together. There was always a split. On one side of the group which comprised people who had been there a long time and were coming out of their madness or whatever it's called, their craziness, being on the verge of moving out. It was a kind of a slum in the house. Their rooms were looked after, they brought flowers into their rooms sometimes, into the kitchen, they cooked meals, and you could either cook your own or participate in a communal meal. Everything was up for grabs as Ronnie* [Laing] *used to say.*

I had to adjust in a house which turned day into night and night into day. So breakfast was around lunch or maybe after lunch … maybe 2pm or 3pm. It was then people got up and started moving around the house; some silent, some chatty, and then life started to warm up around 5pm or 6pm where lunch would get cooked. Dinner was sometime around 10.30pm to 11pm. So my whole structure of time and rhythm was turned not quite upside-down but turned around – that's the concept of autorhythmia, we could follow our own rhythm. There were some timetables given; yoga 2pm, pottery, etc. were offered.

There were some other activities which we would go to; public lectures done by Ronnie [Laing] and other PA members at the Roundhouse. So that was quite a nice thing to do. So there was quite a lot of activity going on.

The house meetings were not compulsory but there was always a lot of double binding going on. There was the house therapists coming to the house and they were getting paid very little. The general agenda of the meetings was first, finances, living together, and chores. Finances were always an issue as was food. Because some people were using more than others, one had to fight for one's rights and stand up to one's own position.

One week the meeting was held at another house and the next week it was held at our house. So it was held at alternative houses each week. There was a feeling of being part of a large community which also felt very nice.

Day-to-day life was actually night-to-night life because people would warm up around 6pm and come to the kitchen which was the centre. This was the centre in most houses, the kitchen or common room. We had a piano and drums in the common room then. We often sat in there as there [were] big windows in that room and light could come in. It was very congenial. But in the evening there was some warmth and discussion and sometimes arguments; lots of smoking ... lots of smoking and endlessly drinking and debates and imagination ... and Ronnie [Laing] this and Ronnie that ... and (another house therapist) this ... So it was a kind of identification process going on. Some people were more open or closed or congenial than others. Also the sexuality in the house between people – that was very much tabooed for a while and I realised, not until I had a relationship with a woman in the house. She was so attractive for me but also very ill. We had a good time. But it was an issue, a tabooed issue. Talking about taboos in the PA it was important ... it was difficult, but we were actually free to talk ... to discuss things. But our ethics, the way we were brought up always came into it and it was a struggle basically ... a struggle.

The idea of what is normal and what is abnormal, or what is mad and what is not mad, and the problematic and struggle (of being a resident in a PA house) of what to do with people who do their own thing were explained by Thomas. Again the idea of autorhythmia came up in the conversation.

Thomas: *In the beginning, one thing I experienced, one chap, an American guy who had been living there a long time, he would not say hello or goodbye. So I thought this was very odd so I told him. He said nothing. So I didn't know what he was about. (A house therapist) said, well this is the situation in the house, you don't have to talk to anyone if you don't want to or tell anyone what you are doing or where you are going. You don't have to communicate; there is no need to if you don't feel any desire. So that was the ethics of the houses.*

It was freer to be in a PA house than say in the (another previous non-PA community), which I experienced before and [in the PA house] *there was no staff/patient distinction directly on a day-to-day level. But it was of course clear that people staying there who were training therapists were training therapists and people who were patients were wholly patients – that was clear. But it was also a bit mystifying. (One house therapist) was a mystifyer, (another house therapist) was sometimes a mystifyer about situations; they did not do it for free* [the house therapists]. *They had a market in the house, everybody went to therapy, and there was lots of psychodynamic language from the second generation people.*

Another thing in comparison to other places, there was the autorhythmia. We had not rigid structures except the community meeting. The rest was up for grabs. One could of course if one went to meeting, one would not turn up late.

But in the house there was nothing set and of course in the (non-PA community where Thomas lived for a period of time previously) everybody cooked, shopped, and participated. In the PA there were also drawing classes and yoga. So there were some structure and time, but generally it was very free. For some people it was more helpful to have a clear structure and for some people it was clear to have very little structure, and very little support. I mean some people were really begging for support and asking for support. Of course one had to own up to one's own voice.

Generally the houses were very nice houses to live in. Sometimes we tried to do a clean-up of communal space or do a bit of gardening, but generally they were not very enticing places to be in. But the (previous non-PA community where Thomas lived) used to have very nice houses. They were better kept so in the chaos there was more room in the (previous non-PA community where Thomas lived) while in the PA the inner chaos was in the outer chaos and it influenced the inner chaos.

Thomas meant that the houses in themselves were nice houses; construction, space, and location etc, but that the living conditions in some of them could become quite un-enticing. The struggle of how to deal with one's assumptions was something that Thomas felt was very helpful in finding one's own feet in the house. Further, unlike orthodox ideas of what helps the psyche flourish, Thomas brought up the idea of humour and having fun together (therapists and residents) as helpful, albeit within a very unorthodox atmosphere which, compared to today's conservative and hyper-regulated standards of how one would look after people in such an establishment, would be unthinkable.

Thomas: *I also found helpful that I was challenged in the house in regards my own inner assumptions about how to live a good life and how to live together and see and be in doubt and to enlarge my tolerance, my ability to be tolerant.*

So that's what I found helpful. Also the humour and the fun we had together in the house like when Ronnie [Laing] came round after the therapy meeting was over, he made a contribution of whisky and he would join in and drink and smoke hashish. So that was part of the ritual when the big master would come round. We would have great fun and a celebration. He would talk a bit and sometimes he would show especially after his daughter died, he would come to the house very sad and he was showing how we can use the households and we can express ourselves in when we are in dire straits in moments in our lives. Showing; that's what Ronnie [Laing] did and I appreciated that.

Of course it was not all rosy in the PA house for Thomas. There were aspects that he found unhelpful.

Thomas: *... the lack of a daily structure, the lack of a daily ritual, the lack of real presence of therapists in the house, of giving a certain hold and warmth in the house. It was left to the inhabitants of the house who were left more or less crazy and mad. The crazier one was, the more attention you got from the house therapists which I thought was curious and interesting to look into. I found this unhelpful. Not everyone was as mad as they tried to be! I also found unhelpful the mystification of the house therapists ... (One house therapist) once said to me that he was just a visitor to the house where ... that I did not find helpful;*

he clearly was the house therapist. So there was this certain triple bind of being inauthentic ... but that was part of the deal ... we always have more aspects to ourselves than we proclaim, or the technique of not to have a technique ... because most people work with a technique like working psychoanalytically and not really being trained psychoanalytically, like (one house therapist). It was really freestyle psychoanalysis because they were hanging around with Ronnie [Laing] or (another PA therapist), so that was not helpful.

Nevertheless, the offer of help was always there, which seemed to be available from some people, and which was perhaps beyond the remit of their role as a house therapist. Again such offers of help/companionship would perhaps be frowned upon today.

Thomas: *Part of what I found helpful was the clarity which I got from (a PA house therapist) who was for me the only one who besides Ronnie [Laing], who I could always approach and make an appointment with if I wanted to. (The PA house therapist) said my door is always open; you can come by if you need some help, please approach me and speak things out. So I found this very good. So he became my elder brother in a sense but also sometimes I found him to be more like a father figure.*

The importance of struggle against one's own demons was an important aspect of why Thomas found the house helpful.

Thomas: *I received what I wanted from the houses. I could go through my depressive moments. I was no bipolar, I was melancholic. I was just prone to depression and being sanguine. When I was melancholic I tended to have rages so I was sometimes bottling up feelings and I would sometimes scream and shout ... I had to really to confront my dark side and accept it.*

Thomas did have some ideas of how the PA houses could have been improved as a result of his experience of being a resident in the PA house.

Thomas: *One could have more houses that were more congenial, in a sense more beautiful. Ronnie [Laing] also liked that – a bit warmer houses, good contacts with the neighbourhood, a bit more structure which came into the PA houses.*

The houses now are completely different compared to the houses we were in – so have a bit more structure. Basically [they] have half the house therapists living in or a community therapist or training therapist living in the house for a while and being present always helps because one could show by experience and show by just being present in the house to share the capabilities and abilities of everydayness. So that is what I would recommend. A bit more structure and clear structures, not mystifying structures which were always there as well, power structures for example, the whole thing about one-upmanship, second to none. All this power struggle which was very 'male-ish'. More yin-yang would be very nice. Of course there was a heyday of eight houses.

What I missed was the supported and guided regression that Winnicott talks about. Sometimes I felt I was regressing in certain moments and difficulties in a session and then going through this in the household and if I had not been able to talk this through with (the PA house therapist) for example I would have been out on a limb and some people were and they were very disappointed because they thought they could come to the house, go down ... you know the Mary Barnes journey into madness and come back up and be more together; some people call this the shamanic journey. Not everyone could be a shaman or return wiser than before the house. Some people were as crazy, sorry to say ... there was some large stupidity which we bring with ourselves of course; stupidity of daily living, phronesis, the wisdom of daily life was not always achieved. Now you can't blame anyone except oneself to be bored ... sometimes it was very boring living in the house day to day, but for me being a student and participant observer and being into anthropology ... it was really good.

I have good thoughts about the PA. It's enriching, its struggling, and its engagement. Laing was very present and playful and we had parties and being together in the community as students, members and residents, and challenging.

BS: Would you recommend the experience of living in the house for people living with mental distress?

Thomas: *Yes of course and also with the assessment. I would have an assessment. People would come to an open door and be seen by someone in the PA and be recommended to one of the houses. I would recommend this to be another person with mental distress. Some people were on medication, some people were off medication. There were some people who had medication and homeopathy. (One PA therapist) I think was a homeopath and he was also a GP; that was helpful. Some people used hash, LSD, mushrooms, but if someone comes to the PA with real mental distress, she or he needs a good guide and should be really, as I felt, attached to a therapist who also could come to the house if need be, even if he or she is not a house therapist and see this person through this so there is a continuation of being guided by a therapist.*

Not for everyone I must say [the PA houses]. *If one could have the PA the way it is now, or the way it was in the past one could say maybe go to different houses which catered for different kinds of people, to see what they are like. We had this; houses catering for different types of people and distress and we also had different types of therapists in the different houses. Sometimes there was more Jungian, more humanist, especially the re-birthing thing and we went to re-birthing workshops. Some people could not take it, but I would recommend it with those provisions.*

BS: Are the alternatives to the houses any better or worse?

Thomas: *Well I don't know about now, but in my time in comparison to the PA and (the other non-PA community where Thomas had lived) it was sometimes better and sometimes worse and compared to the therapeutic communities of Maxwell Jones and the communities set up after the '59 Act* [The Mental Health Act of 1959] *in different areas of England … sometimes Arbours* [another organisation which runs communities], *some people were better off in Arbours; they had a very clear structure.*

But for me, for patients I have known, we found it was magic in a way to live in the PA house, to have an alternative and understanding to mental distress or the spiritual aspects of suffering. There was a basic humour. But it is a pity [that the following reform did not happen] *that Ronnie* [Laing] *and (another PA member) tried to push reform in the PA into a bit more of an integrative approach; bio-therapy, a warm, humble and spiritual approach, like a monastery, music, meditation, martial arts. (Another PA therapist) suggested this to Ronnie* [Laing]. *But to have these approaches, open and more clear; not mystifying, but still able to name things, not just psychoanalysis and phenomenology. Demystified houses!*

They are doing a good service for people and I think it is exciting to continue the work and to have houses and have clarity, and also a certain humbleness and not be mystifying. To not have double/treble binds. It was not always psychoanalytical or phenomenological; that was only one aspect. There was the mythological; the village of healers!

Endnotes

1. Mary Barnes was an English artist and writer who suffered from schizophrenia but recovered to become a successful painter. She is particularly known for her documentation of her experience at R.D. Laing's experimental therapeutic community, Kingsley Hall, London. This account is published in *Two Accounts of a Journey through Madness* (2002) with Joseph Berke, published by Other Press.
2. A description of the film from the Kino Lorber website (www.kinolorber.com/video.php?id=697). 'In 1971, filmmaker Peter Robinson and a small crew entered a world of anarchic madness and healing compassion unlike any other. The resulting film, *Asylum*, records their seven-week stay in radical psychiatrist R.D. Laing's controversial Archway Community – a London row-house where the inmates literally run the asylum. Laing's conviction that schizophrenics can only heal their shattered "self" where they're free and yet are held responsible for their actions, challenged patients, doctors and, in *Asylum*'s incredible document, the filmmakers, to live communally and peacefully.'

Chapter Fifteen

David

David is another ex-resident of the PA houses who had had previous admissions to a psychiatric hospital. He came to get in touch with the PA when after the second hospital admission he was in 'dire straits'. His story is quite a remarkable one.

BS: How did you hear about the houses?

David: *I was, had been hospitalised for a combination of (psychiatric disorders). So I actually heard via my psychiatrist. It was a slightly informal connection. I think the senior social worker, he worked with my psychiatrist and happened to know one of the PA house therapists so I think she was aware of the house through that and got a contact number through that. I got the number through that, but it took me a wee while to follow it up. I did not do it after my first stay in hospital but after my second when I was discharged when I was really in dire straits I got in touch.*

After getting in touch with the PA David had to go to four or five house meetings. What is striking about these meetings is the lack of formal psychiatric diagnosis, enquiry, or risk assessment that would be the case in most institutions dealing with people with 'mental health' difficulties or mental distress.

BS: What was the purpose of those initial meetings? How were they run? What was talked about in them?

David: *There was never any clear focus or agenda. I mean partly it was people asking me about myself, but it was also people talking about issues that they were having in the house and there was a lot of stuff between how different people in the house were getting on. Quite a lot around conflict resolution. Obviously there were a lot of problematic relationships in the house. Yeah a lot of tension around that and a large part of that was what was talked about.*

David was sympathetic to the 'therapeutic' ideology of the PA and had experienced psychotherapy and counselling before, although this had been unhelpful for him.

BS: Had you had experience of psychotherapy before?

David: *Yeah, I had had individual psychotherapy before; about two to three years which I had not found particularly helpful. But I suppose I was broadly sympathetic to the idea of therapy and counselling by then as I don't think I would have wanted to come into the house otherwise. It was obvious that therapy was a very big part of the whole setup.*

BS: Did they encourage you to be in your own individual therapy?

David: *They did yes. It took a long time before that was started. I think the first year I was barely managing physically and emotionally I felt under a great deal of stress although it was still vastly preferable to living with my parents; that was completely intolerable. The house was though a very difficult place to live. I found it very hard living there … My ability to get out was quite limited as well. So it was quite some time before I started seeing a therapist and that somebody was not a PA therapist but was somebody that one of the house therapists knew. He turned out to be very good actually. I certainly benefited a lot from seeing him.*

Like many of the PA houses, three, four or even five meetings per week were common. This again was stressful according to accounts given by David.

David: *It was very difficult … I think and if you were around they would expect you to go to the meetings and if you did not people would wonder why you were not there. There was quite a lot of peer pressure and from the therapists to attend as many meetings as possible. Many years later I decided that it was probably overkill. I think more than three per week is more than anyone can reasonably put up with in a week. So it was very hard. I was doing my very best to follow that regime but I found it incredibly difficult, stressful and quite exhausting. The meetings themselves were often quite fraught. There was a lot of going on about I suppose quite trivial things, quite little things between people that would get talked about and more often than not I felt they were getting escalated rather than any sort of light being shed upon what was going on. At the same time there was a feeling of emotional connection between us, so there was a sense of us being part of something even though we were at each other's throats. I think there was a sense of intimacy there. We did all talk about very difficult and painful things from our pasts as well in quite an open manner which I think did lead us into a connection between us. But there were also the discussions about the practicalities of keeping a house, sharing a house. Sharing a house is not the easiest thing to do at the best of times and especially so with people who are suffering considerable mental distress. So a fair amount of the meetings were taken up with that which was often quite helpful …*

… One drawback of the house I found was that because there were too many meetings and there was such an emphasis on the meetings, sometimes people were reluctant to sort things out between themselves informally and so disputes and issues that might usually be resolved in a fairly everyday way were getting held over to the next meeting and getting talked about at the meetings. Sometimes the energy would have gone or you know the situation would have moved on and it was sometimes a bit stilted. Not always, sometimes it could be very useful discussions about conflict and need, but I think the sheer number of meetings meant that there was a slight tendency for more of us to do that [hold things in mind for the meetings rather than resolve informally outside the meetings]. *I think also perhaps we were all quite anxious people as a result of our various experiences and situations. I think sometimes we were just scared of conflict and scared to engage in potential conflict situations if there was not the reassuring presence of the therapist there.*

BS: So it sounds like a kind of bottling-up process that could go on?

David: *Yeah.*

In terms of what was helpful during his stay in the houses, David highlighted the struggle and helpfulness of being challenged.

BS: In terms of your own distress you were going through, what was helpful for you?

David: *I was challenged. I think it gave me an opportunity to see very young childish parts of myself which I think I was quite ashamed of and not very much in touch with and quite resistant to exploring But they obviously played themselves out* [with] *other people in the house. That was something that was brought up in the meetings. So although I found that difficult and painful, I think it was quite helpful. I talked a lot about relationships. That was my difficulty with personal relationships, especially sexual relationships with the opposite sex. That was something that was a big difficulty for me. It was good to talk with other people who experienced the same difficulties as well. I think I found that enormously helpful; to talk about relationships and sex and those sorts of things. I found that very, very helpful;* [having] *very deep, intimate, and quite profound conversations with people in and out of the meetings, which I found enormously uplifting. I mean first of all, just the process of just acknowledging just how crap inside I really did feel, which took a while because I was quite well defended I think. But in a fairly kind of sophisticated way. Then having acknowledged that it was very useful for me to realise that pretty much we are all in the same boat. The symptoms and the ways it affected our lives … I think we* [David and the other residents] *were very different as individuals, our personalities were all very different. But I think there was an underlying understanding. Something we* [David and the other residents] *have all shared in common as well which I found very helpful. I found the presence of the therapists very helpful as well. They were both very experienced and very compassionate people. I think they were certainly saner than my parents were. They didn't do my head in the same way that my parents did. They certainly did do my head in at times. I was never uncritical in my discussions with them but yeah, they helped enormously. They were role models to us to a certain extent, certainly to begin with.*

David came to his 'own mind' about what was beneficial for him and was able to evaluate his experiences of the PA house that reminded me

of Montaigne's essay '*On Experience*' (Montaigne, 1991), an essay that inspired R.D. Laing and the subsequent founding of the PA and its houses. Montaigne encouraged people to come to their 'own mind' in the trials of the human condition and not rely on advice by experts to tell one how to live one's life. David also made some important contrasts between other kinds of care for those in mental distress and where he was after his experience of living in a PA house.

David: *I think therapy is a bit like vitamins. In small doses I think they can be very useful. I think if you have too much it becomes poisonous. I think we did have too much. There were too many meetings. There was an ethos of sorts of sorting everything out through the meetings and one did kind of lose a grip on everyday life. I mean there was only seven of us there I think; I think one person was working, one person was studying. The rest of us, myself included, were pretty much incapacitated. I think there was not enough focus on rehab at the same time as therapy. I think there was an idea that we sort ourselves out until we are ready to go out into the world rather than the therapy is there to help us as we get into the world. I think that was the problem. And I think those who got the best out of it were those that were quite critical and never saw therapy as this great sort of saviour. We never completely believed in therapy as the therapists did and some of the other house members did, but we made use of it. We did all become terribly introspective. I remember it took me about a year after I moved out of the house to get over that and kind of learn how to relate to people. There was a certain re-conditioning and we did get institutionalised, probably much less than if we had been in hospital or some kind of long-term psychiatric treatment. I don't want to do the house down, but nevertheless there was a bit of institutionalism that did take place and the longer one was there, the more pronounced that became. For about a year I had to sort of de-condition myself after the house.*

BS: I understand what you mean about being too immersed in therapy … my partner often tells me to stop talking like a therapist!

(Both laugh)

David: *I think that was it. I think having learned to question ourselves and reflect in a way that was very helpful; we then had to learn when not to do that and how to be ordinary. I think probably that was one of the drawbacks of being immersed in therapy.*

BS: That's what I was going to say. You did say that you have had hospital admissions as well. Compared to a hospital environment what was the house experience like?

David: *Vastly superior. I have been quite critical I think partly because if the houses are to survive and to flourish I would genuinely like to see them do that. I think it is important to see how they can do things better. But I suppose partly I am coming from the perspective of what the ideal house could be. However, when you compare the houses to, and I have had a fair amount of experience of this as well, the medical model, medication-based approach to mental illness, there is no doubt the houses are far superior. It would be, in terms of what I have said today, it would be tragic if the baby was thrown out with the bath water. I think the basic ... I mean to me the houses prove that the medical model ... you know I have never believed the medical model of mental health. I never believed it was analogous to having high blood pressure or something like that; so you take pills the rest of your life for bipolar disorder or schizophrenia or whatever. I have never bought into that analogy. But I also think the house proved* [its effectiveness], *because I was a wreck when I went in there. I can't really express just what terrible shape physically* [I was in]; *the reality was it was entirely due to psychological factors. It was entirely by addressing the psychological factors in the house and in my own therapy and yes in life outside, as I have carried on doing, that my physical condition improved ... I think the house therapists were extremely helpful in linking explicitly to my psychology and not letting me off the hook on that issue. As a result I improved enormously and there is no doubt the basic process worked and you know I would be ... I don't really see how I could have managed without something like that. And I think hospital is appalling. I couldn't live with my parents, I could not be in hospital. Yes it was very different living in the house and I have a number of suggestions (laughs) in which it could be made easier, but it was still a hell of a lot better than any of the alternatives available that I know of. And I am quite passionate about the potential of what the houses can, could and should do. I think they are enormously helpful things. I do want to support them even though I had my difficulties there as I have said.*

Some moving last words from David.

David: *I feel as though I have utterly transcended the situation that I was in when I went into the house. That is also partly due to my own efforts since I came out the house, but that made it possible for me to get onto that foothold. So the house has taken me out of the NHS care altogether.*

Chapter Sixteen

Peter

Peter is a man who stayed in one of the early PA community houses. As has been documented by Laing (see Mullan, 1995), this was a period (the 1960s and 1970s) of great experimentation and a journey into the unknown. Many who flocked to the early PA communities were drawn there by the work of R.D. Laing.

Peter: *I guess I wrote to Ronnie* [Laing] *in the winter of (19XX). I told him I was finishing my studies at university and I would like to come to meet him, and he said in a letter in the post, 'Come to London and join the dance'. That was his words. When I arrived in London I lived with a friend in (London) and I met him* [Laing] *and Aaron Esterson at the time and within a short time Ronnie said 'Why don't you come and stay with us in the community?' He explained to me a little bit of how it worked. So I moved in within the next day or two. I did not have a flat or room or anything, so I took my luggage and I moved in. That was how that happened. I had a good chat to Ronnie once in his consulting room about what I was doing and what I thought. I had been reading the books* The Self and Others *and* The Divided Self. *There wasn't the other book at the time … The Politics of Experience. It was in the making So there was not a lot, but I liked his approach and also it felt like I was being part of something that was exciting. It felt like anything was possible. Things had been stagnating for years* [in society] *but in the PA house nothing was fixed, there were no rules, it was up to the people who lived there to work out what to do. There was no authority there except the level of consciousness of the people. The person with the greatest authority was the person who had the greatest consciousness of what was going on.*

So that was how I heard about (the PA community house). My motivation was that I wanted to find out what it was all about and I wanted to be close to Ronnie and to hear him talk and find out what was going on. It seemed like a really great opportunity ... so ...

The lack of a formal 'therapeutic or psychiatric structure' in the PA community house, which was a response to what Laing saw as the existing abusive psychiatric system, was evident during the interview with Peter.

Peter: *Well, in terms of therapy, there was no ongoing therapy except there were a few people that Ronnie saw* [in his private practice]. *He did not see any people in the building itself. He was against having what it is called now; a house therapist.*

BS: Really?

Peter: *He didn't want people there because they were therapists. He wanted people who loved the ideas. He* [Ronnie] *said it was probably better if there were no doctors or psychologists here at all. He said he would have preferred if there were carpenters and washer women; these kinds of people had knowledge of human life and a love of people. That would be great he* [Ronnie] *said. But unfortunately a lot of people who were into psychology wanted to be there because they thought they would learn something, or maybe become famous ...*

... So that was my experience. Day-to-day life was what it was all about. So the therapy, I mean as someone often said, therapy is not something that should be consigned to the consulting room. Therapy is going on all the time in one form or another, in one's life. So one shouldn't think it is a professional activity necessarily. It is the way the soul is met with by other people. Some ways are very destructive and devastating, other ways are the opposite ...

... As we got more people, there used to be up to fifteen or sixteen people living there and people would come to stay a couple of nights on sleeping bags on the floor of the games room and then they would go again. So we had a lot of movement. It was open to people coming for short times. Other people might have written from abroad. There were a couple of people whose parents wrote

from India, the children were living in London. Somehow or other people came searching for help from a lot different places and would meet Ronnie first of all and then Ronnie would let the people who were living in the building decide who they wanted to stay.

BS: Were these people who came to live in the house primarily people who had mental health problems?

Peter: *Yes, of course. It was (the PA community house) well known for being an alternative. In Ronnie's words it was an 'asylum'. Which is a very nice word, but it has connotations as being some kind of crazy house. The neighbours down the road from (the PA community house) … they used to write with sticks of chalk on the front door of (the PA community house) 'nuthouse' and 'crazy house'.*

BS: Really!?

Peter: *And break the windows by throwing rocks and bricks so the place became quite draughty. We would get wind howling through, nobody had the time to fix the windows, it took skill and art and we did not have the equipment. There was nothing to do except wait until somebody came to repair them. So it was a bit like, well it was an asylum … It was a shelter, it was a rundown* [place] … *It was like a space ship from another time. There were many passengers. You could try anything – as Ronnie often said, 'There are no rules here except you are not allowed to attack anybody, smash things, break things, or act dangerous.' There were very few rules.*

There were big differences between the psychiatric hospital and the PA community house (where Peter stayed) in the way mental distress was viewed. Such an approach is today a part of the ethos of the PA house, although in the community house Peter stayed in, it was perhaps more extreme or radical.

Peter: *… Ronnie would say, sometimes joking at first, 'We all need to learn to be a bit more mad.' He encouraged people who were there* [in the PA house] *who were not suffering or diagnosed with something, to just let go, to let their* own madness come out. He did not say, 'do and say mad crazy things', but 'just try to let go a bit'. We were all against electroshock at the time. I visited a mental hospital once and interviewed the consultant psychiatrist and he told me sitting across from him at his desk how he performed lobotomies and how you have to be careful because it's only a small part of the brain one is operating on with a scalpel. Only one slip of a couple of millimetres and you can out a whole wrong portion of the brain. And we knew that and we knew the results of electroshock. It was widely used; I am not sure about today.

BS: Oh yes, you can still get electroshock today.

Peter: *There was a feeling amongst us that we could speak about it. There was something to struggle against in society, a collective thing; we were working so to change things.*

The topic of psychiatric medication came up in the interview. It is often thought that the ethos of the early PA community where Peter stayed was completely against psychiatric medication of all kinds and use. However, such a totalitarian system did not actually exist.

Peter: *Quite a few people who came to (the PA community house) had come from a mental hospital and their psychiatrists had been giving them Largactil, Stelazine or something similar like that. They were meant to be taking the stuff; usually they would not bother after a while, but some of them had to report after a while* [to their psychiatrist] *so they had to keep taking their drugs. There was not as much enforcement as there is today. It was a bit more lax. If you were not dangerous, you were left* [alone] *so Ronnie never prescribed medication at all. I think sometimes he would give someone a tranquilliser if the person was in a lot of distress but it was not the policy of the place. It was not an either/or, he was just saying why do we have to make people take drugs when they can get along with human contact? There was a lot of love at (the PA community house). A lot of caring and I think that Ronnie showed people that he cared by the way that he treated people, how he dealt with them … he was a Scotsman, he had a real temper, but he also had a huge sense of humour and a love of music. I mean music for him was so essential. (Another resident), who was a resident from* somewhere else [another PA community], *came to (our PA community house) and played Chopin on the piano and Ronnie also played Chopin and Beethoven. Ronnie also loved jazz. He would even join us in dancing. He had his own style of dancing; he would just do his own style. People loved him being around and joining in. There was a feeling of community and I think that says a lot really.*

BS: So are you saying the ethos was one of anti-medication; were people encouraged by people like Ronnie and yourself to come off medication?

Peter: *Oh I would encourage somebody if there was any possibility that they could do without it. I might say, 'Why don't you see, try it out.' Ronnie might have said the same thing. There was no policy as such like 'you should be on medication or you should not be', in those days. There was no kind of issue ... Loren Mosher died recently. He set up communities in California. He was a really good guy. He was totally against medication for mental health and the psychopharmaceutical industry. He said that the American Psychiatric Association should change its name to the American Psychopharmaceutical Association.*

Peter then went on to describe a situation at his PA community house which depicted how people would deal with a crisis with a fellow resident. Peter helped out in a way that in today's climate would seem quite unconventional.

Peter: *There was a time when a girl from America, she was living in (a city) and she had (X number of) children and she had quite a lot of money and she was living on her own in (a city) and she had a boyfriend. After reading a bit of Ronnie's work she wanted to find out what schizophrenia was all about. So she decided to eat a gram of hash a day. So she did this and she went completely out of it. And she did not come down either. So she flew over to London and she had an appointment to see Ronnie. She was in analysis for a short time with him. One night Ronnie came up to (the PA community house), it was quite late; it must have been after 9pm. He said, 'I am going to send a lady to you, she would like to come to (the PA community house), if you could see her and find her a room that would be great.' Well she did not come till after midnight. She came in a taxi, got out of the taxi and came into the building. She was really raving.*

She was in about her (her approximate age) and very articulate in some ways. She was talking to some voices in the ceiling, which were her boyfriend and some other people. She was addressing them and then she would address me and … She did not want to sleep and she was up for four days.

BS: Four days!?

Peter: *In which I had to follow her around. I was trying to keep track of her in case she harmed herself. She was not a harm to other people but she could have harmed herself. So after four days she finally gave up and went to sleep. That was Audrey* [a fictitious name]. *Later her parents took a private plane from (a country) to see her in London. Ronnie was going to meet them in (the PA community house). He did not know what the meeting was going to be about and he was going to ask this woman to be there with her parents, and he was not sure how it was going to go* [the meeting]. *I had heard Audrey or Ronnie say that she had thought about taking Largactil* [a psychiatric drug] *for that day or something and I said to her, 'If you are frightened of this stuff I'll take some with you, be your companion if you like.' So I took it and I felt awful. It cuts you off like you're in cotton wool, you don't feel anything, you can't speak, you can't think, you're just in a daze. Hopeless stuff. That was my one experience of Largactil. Anyway, that was one of the difficult people. There are several people I could talk about who were really difficult, there were people who got real benefit out of the place, people who misused it or were destructive.*

Peter then went on to describe how there were many activities that went on at his PA community house that are not part of today's PA houses.

Peter: *… We sometimes had three to five people* [in a theatre group] *and we made up exercises which I had learned from (a theatre group) … I think they were based in Paris or New York and they travelled round the world and they did very mythological things. They performed in the Roundhouse in Camden … Ronnie also told me to read a book by Frances Yates* [Giordano Bruno and the Hermetic Tradition]. *In that book I learned about Marsilio Ficino for the first time. But there were also books around about yoga. Ronnie encouraged me and others to do yoga and meditate together. We would meet early in the morning* *every day for a while. We would sit cross-legged in the meditation room. Ronnie would love to meditate because he was heavily into meditation.*

BS: So it was more than just the idea of psychotherapy that you sit in a room in a one to one. There were the arts and the theatre; there was physical activity, yoga, meditation. It was a very holistic setup.

Peter: *There was no programme. In terms of one's own imagination and intuition, in terms of what would be good to do. People were drawn because of the people who did it. If they wanted to be a part of something happening they might come and do yoga for a while or do meditation, or they might stay in their room.*

The idea of 'going down', letting somebody go down into their madness, and the questioning of madness was something that Laing and Peter's PA community house encouraged.

BS: Talking about going down, Thomas Merton and the book written by St John of the Cross, *The Dark Night of the Soul*, they both talk about going down.[1]

Peter: *This was the one thing that was probably of uppermost importance for* [the ethos of PA community experience]. *Ronnie understood this very well, the importance of this. He had experienced this as a young psychiatrist of having two or three patients described in the book* Wisdom, Madness and Folly. *They were young men who were in a mental hospital … so he invited them to come to his house and stay with his family. It was very daring and very courageous thing to do. So he had experience of somebody going to their room, going down and being quiet. For him, when he* [Ronnie] *visited the padded cells in the mental hospital, he would try to get them to calm down and talk, and usually they would be fine with him sitting in the padded cell; which was something nobody had done before. So in many ways my image of Ronnie was of that really like Pinel who was a French psychiatrist who must have been the first psychiatrist who took the chains off the patients who were chained to the wall. Ronnie was the first person who wanted to take away the drugs … and find out what was going on. The first thing he ever said, I think the first dinner time at (the PA community house), or one of the first ... He went around the table and said, 'I wonder if everybody sitting around who is here tonight could tell of their experience of madness, watching someone else go through it, or having gone through it themselves?' Everybody talked at the table and some interesting things came out of it.*

The idea that getting to grips with mental distress and working with those in mental distress was more than just a job, as it is generally considered in many sectors of the mental health industry, but a calling, became evident from Peter's description of his stay at his PA community house.

BS: Do you think the wounded healer idea was present at (the PA community house)?

Peter: *I think Laing would have certainly understood it. The thing about Chiron, are of the stories of him in his later life. Heracles had found that Prometheus had been taken by Zeus and chained to the mountainside where the vultures were eating his liver every day and it was growing back. He was in constant pain and agony. Zeus said that he would never let him away from his suffering, which Prometheus had brought on himself by disobeying his orders. However, Zeus said to Chiron that if he found somebody to take the place of Prometheus then he would let him go. Chiron agreed to go in his place and became chained and had the horrible experience. He actually accepted to die and to go into Hades. He was sent after he dies to Zeus. Zeus raised him up to be a constellation in the sky. Hillman[2] says that the archetype of the wounded healer is split into two. Usually in psychotherapy you have the wounded person and the healer. So they are sitting across from each other. They don't see that they are actually one archetype and when they are split like that the one person gets all the energy and the transference of being healed, the other one wrecked and ruined and mad whatever. Whatever he or she does he can never find a way to be equal to that person. So it is split, and Hillman thinks that's a big shame.*

BS: That's like modern day psychiatry. They regard themselves as healers and in a very medical sense: 'I am the doctor, healer or psychotherapist, and you are sick.'

Peter: *But that's it. The experience of having gone through some form of breakdown or madness, Ronnie would have recognised it as a very important background experience for someone who was going to come and stay at (the PA community house). He would have honoured and respected that ... and he would have actually encouraged people going through their madness to go down, like Mary Barnes did. The whole argument with Esterson was over the fact that Ronnie was backing Mary to go down, saying it was alright. Ronnie used to say in our society you are encouraged always to progress, to go forward, sometimes you are allowed to go sideways, but never to go backwards, you can't regress; regression is not allowed.*

BS: Yes, it is very success orientated, our culture. Were there many people at (the PA community house) who recognised this idea? I read about Leon Redler and Steve Gans in their book *Just Listening*; they talked about their own struggles, going through stuff, so I suppose a lot of people who came to (the PA community house) must have recognised there was a place for them, you know the attempt to try to rejoin the split archetype of the wounded healer in some respect. And do you see that for yourself as well?

Peter: *Oh yes, alchemically. I would say that alchemically I experienced the nigredo.*[3] *I was going through a lot of difficult stuff, so to go somewhere for this to happen, to feel that I was part of something, the value of this type of experience was recognised. So some people who came there to work might have become quite superior, which the guy I mentioned earlier* [a therapist who worked at Peter's PA community house], *he became quite superior minded I think. Whereas, some people* [residents and people involved with the PA community house] *became quite cynical with what they saw, people misusing, abusing the place, but to develop a nuance you have to see what is the misuse and what they are actually doing. You've got to point it out to them and get them to see their shadow or their aspect of their Nafs* [a Sufi term for egotistical behaviour]. *They have to see what they are doing which is causing distress or destruction, something about them that can't be criticised, about what they can't take criticism for, get them to see that they see that their way is the right way, but they are blind to the fact that they are being cruel, destructive, and mean.*

Testimony of experience

Peter was quite pessimistic regarding the progress that had been made since the days of his stay in a PA community house in regards how people in mental distress are generally thought about.

BS: I would like to know why in today's society, do you think there is a place in society for the likes of a PA community house you stayed in or today's PA houses (which are a bit different from the early PA community house you stayed in), and do you think there is a place today for the experience that you and others went through at your PA community house, or do you think psychiatry is still far off the track?

Peter: *There certainly is a huge place* [for the ethos of the PA communities] *but I don't think there is room being made, a place where that could be. Theoretically it is a very important place to happen, but it is not as if we have progressed from those ideas of that time. I don't think people have advanced that much in their ideas about the psyche. Laing was always trying to understand what madness was and how it came about. He was not trying just to treat it. So how have we progressed scientifically? So we now work with DNA and the reasons why someone is diagnosed schizophrenic, do we figure out what is wrong with our DNA so we can correct it? The genetic argument, Laing replied to many times, but the thing is statistically it* [the DNA hypothesis of mental illness] *does not hold water, but they keep bringing it up ... So we have not progressed in the sense of a linear line; going in one direction. I mean primitive societies, we have learned how they should progress, how to become more civilised, how to become like us, how to have television, telephones, machinery. Somehow this thought has replaced a lot of mythological thought which was part of ancient societies which was put together very beautifully. That has been replaced with a very shallow form of scientism ...*

... So to come back to that question about what would happen now and is there a place for the ethos of a place like (the PA community house), I think some kind of, call it a revolution, a very large change in society on a collective level is needed, because individually private institutions, they will be stamped out and stopped like somebody starting up the school like Summerhill.[4] *They are being fought on every level by education departments to shut the place down, even*

though the place is good and the teaching is wonderful. So if somebody shows that a 'community' has many good things it may still be shut down for some reason; say because people may be frightened or threatened You will have to involve parliament for a change to occur. The way the media is going it is taking over as the 'thought police' as we used to call it in the 60s. They have greater and greater power. If people see how much they are being controlled and if somebody speaks out, they are made to think they don't see reality.

Endnotes

1. Thomas Merton (1915–1968) was an Anglo-American Catholic, a prolific writer and student of mysticism of many religious and spiritual traditions. St John of the Cross (1542–1591) was a major figure of the Counter-Reformation, a Spanish mystic, a Roman Catholic saint, a Carmelite friar and a priest who was born at Fontiveros, Old Castile. One of his most famous works was *The Dark Night of the Soul.* In this work he discussed the mystical practice of being with one's Dark Night, instead of trying to escape from it. These two writers and mystics have much to offer in regard to the human condition, mental distress and how to cope and live with them. Their respective wisdoms are contrary to medico-scientific methods of dealing with mental distress.

2. James Hillman (1926–2011) was an American psychologist. He studied at, and then guided studies for, the C.G. Jung Institute in Zurich, founded a movement towards archetypal psychology, and retired into private practice, writing and travelling to lecture, until his death at his home in Connecticut.

3. The nigredo, or blackening phase, is a term related to alchemy and the alchemical process of individuation. The nigredo implies a time of depression and mental despair. This time of life feels unfavourable. You feel wretched, caught in a black mood whose foundation may seem difficult to identify. This is because your current ego attitudes are redundant, and due to lack of adaptableness you feel stuck. These feelings may come into your life owing to an overload of stress in daily life. As these feelings

become more unbearable the notion that life is meaningless comes to the fore. It is simply that life as your ego has known it in the past is obsolete. The subconscious begins to revolt, seeking a psychological revolution in attitudes. If you listen to the voice within your depression, you come to realise that you must willingly subject yourself to change.

4. Summerhill School is an independent British boarding school based on A.S. Neill's principle of 'freedom, not licence'. This extends to the freedom for pupils to choose which lessons, if any, they attend.

Chapter Seventeen

Debbie

Like many of the people I talked to, Debbie described the process for getting into a PA house as very informal with little semblance to 'entrance' into most places that house people with mental distress (e.g., a psychiatric hospital).

Debbie: *I just rang up. I had to visit the house however many times to go to the house meetings. It all happened very quickly. I visited four or five times and just moved in.*

BS: What was the nature of the meetings that you went there for?

Debbie: *Just the house meetings where the house therapists and residents meet round the table and talk about the things that are going on. You just go as a visitor and if they want to talk to you they talk to you. If they have got things to talk about they talk about other things. You don't have to join in. You know if they like you, you can stay, if they don't like you, you can't stay. Basically it's up to the people in the house. The therapists can try and persuade. I was on the other end of it obviously when I was in the house, and some people they just didn't like and they didn't get to come basically.*

BS: So a kind of an informal interview type of thing?

Debbie: *Yeah, I guess so yeah. It really wasn't an interview. It was just a suck it and see really if they liked you and you liked them.*

BS: So what were your expectations of the house?

Debbie: *I did not have any expectations, I just hoped that I could live somewhere, you know, I was in a rut, things were not getting any better, so it was just hoping that things got better ... but not really knowing how ... or you know ... knowing there is just nowhere to go. I had tried everything ... I had no other options really ... you just stay miserable and ill, or try something else.*

Debbie had experience of being in psychiatric care but like many of my interviewees this had been of little help.

BS: Did you have any experience of psychiatric care before you went into the house?

Debbie: *Yeah. My main problem was (a psychiatric disorder) and I had been in hospital loads of times and all it really taught me was to stay out of hospital. All I learned was that there was no point in going through that again. I didn't learn anything so I learned to keep myself out of hospital, but I had not learned how to live life so to speak. I just learned how to survive and that's not enough really ... not enough for me anyway. Some people get to that point and they chug along, thinking it can be OK but I think I kind of stayed at that level for quite a few years, not really being well, but not ill enough to be in hospital and, you know, nothing changes. Therapy was OK but even that was not enough and I think the only thing that would have been enough was living with other people.*

Living in a PA house for Debbie was no utopia. As she describes, one has to be ready for the difficulty. Although it was difficult, paradoxically, Debbie found dealing with her difficulties and the difficulties of living in the house positive. The issue of coming to one's own mind when wanting to leave or have a change was evident in the discussion. This is contrary to how most mental health professionals deal with the discharge of 'patients'.

BS: I suppose the big question is what was your overall experience of the house?

Debbie: *Probably for 90 per cent of the time absolutely awful. But then that's how it is – it's a horrible place because you can't run away from it. Basically I think most people find ways of running away from things in their life. In life you* know, you can do that, you can avoid everything if you wanted but in the house unless you leave the house, but don't really want to do that because you have got nowhere really else to go. It's just like being trapped.*

BS: Really?

Debbie: *But in a positive way, in the long run, but it is a kind of trap. I mean you have to be bad enough ... I mean lots of people did leave because they came across things that they found very difficult* [to deal with] *and if you don't want to face them then you just leave and people did leave but maybe that's because they were not desperate enough to go through it. But I think it only works if you are very desperate and you have nowhere else to go . . you know ... that's your option ... to stay and deal with stuff. It's like unless you are at your lowest point it probably won't work, if you still think there are other options that might be easier, then you'll probably leave and that was quite interesting. I saw quite a lot of that. I knew people who thought if I went off and did this or went off there and did that it would be better ... but you ... just living in the house with lots of people, having house meetings every day.*

BS: You said it was like hell?

Debbie: *Yeah, I don't remember it being like that. I saw it as a positive thing. In the last year or so I felt really good. Obviously it helped me in my life. I've got everything I ever wanted and that is purely down to the house, so I have happy thoughts and feelings about it, but most of the time I was living there I had thoughts about it being hell and wanting to leave. But when I was quite ready to leave I wanted to stay! You know when you're happy to stay that's when you're ready to leave.*

BS: Paradoxical?

Debbie: *Completely because you have got nothing to hide from anymore, you've got nothing to run away from anymore.*

BS: What was the most horrible thing about living in the house?

Debbie: *Other people, how I felt about other people, how I felt they felt about me, trying to live alongside other people without making myself disappear, having to relate to other people. I had no idea how to do it, having to deal with my emotions with other people. That's the intellectual version because at the time it just felt like I was scared all the time. There were good moments within that. I guess you have got to have good moments as well otherwise you would not keep going. There were some good times with people that made you think it was worth carrying on. But I think even in the house I would get to the point where I went downhill again and they were flapping their arms around and saying 'what's she doing?' Again, I think it's going to your lowest point and finding a way out of it, finding a new way out of it. My way out of it was to have communal meals which they didn't have when I was there. I think they had them historically. They had them before but they kind of stopped them. And I think that helped everybody actually in the end. It was such a simple thing. It was a pivotal moment sometime I remember when one house therapist said, 'What can we do? We can't seem to do anything to help you, what can we do?' I just said oh ... communal meals because I just couldn't deal with the cooking. I don't think anyone could deal with it really, having to share a kitchen with eight people, cook all the different meals at different times and do the shopping. Obviously for me it was really, really, awful. But it I think helped a lot of people. It certainly helped me have nice meal experiences really which kind of made the whole thing ... kind of changed me really.*

At one point during her stay, the house therapists became very worried for Debbie's physical and mental state.

Debbie: *But maybe I needed people to be worried about me. That's important as well. It's not just the people you live with. It's also your relationship with your therapist, they care for you, they don't just do therapy, they do care about you, and maybe why the houses are so hard because it takes a lot out of the therapists. You know, they* [the house therapists] *always go the extra mile, you kind of learn ... I don't know ... whether I forced them into it or ... I don't know ... you can't really analyse yourself too much can you (laughs). I guess when I look back on it I guess I wanted someone to worry about me or to be upset about me or something. So yeah they were quite worried, but you know they didn't put me in hospital.*

BS: Were they averse to such a move?

Debbie: *Oh yeah, but I think they were worried for my actual physical health, but obviously I don't think they would have anyone in hospital. A few people did end up in hospital if they became very manic. They were not averse to it when it became necessary. But I suppose they would try not to do it. The care you get from the therapists, they were incredibly amazing people who care about you for no reason (laughs) … if you are there for (X amount of) years and you see them every day it's quite a strong bond.*

The ordinariness of day-to-day life, the house meetings, and her perceived ethos of the PA house were discussed by Debbie.

BS: How would you describe the nature of the house meetings?

Debbie: *Just literally, sit down at the table, who said what to whom today, who's got something wrong today, who's depressed. Really very unpredictable, and the talkative people talk, and the quiet people don't talk, and they would try to bring you out if you were quiet. It was very much suck it and see and see what happens on the day. Whoever wanted to talk, talked, but I think if you had not talked for a long time they would question you. For me that is my worst nightmare, having to talk in front of people, you know there were usually seven to eight people there with four therapists.*

BS: Do you think there was a kind of air or ethos surrounding everything?

Debbie: *Anti-drugs, anti-hospital, very … try to give everyone a chance, try to tolerate bad behaviour, anger. It was sometimes a very fine line between being hostile to other people, but you had to try to put up with other people's anger a lot of the time. It was not pleasant. It would either be other people's anger or madness. There were a lot of hard things to deal with. Things were made to be tolerated by the support of the meetings. It was almost like you wouldn't have to tolerate them if you were not in the house, but if you were in the house you had to have support to put up with these things. It was a bit of a vicious circle. Sometimes you would think what if this person was not so mad then you wouldn't need to have all these meetings. So I guess that was the whole point of being in the house is that it has mad people in it. We all had our own madness and we all had to put up with each other, which is really hard, which I think is part of the hardness I think. That is that you are in a vulnerable position and ideally you would like some nice warm cosy place to live and be protected and it was completely the opposite. You had more to deal with than most people. I came out of it fine, but I think some people found it pretty distressing and maybe did not ... I can't talk for others ... I guess it has the potential to be quite damaging, people can be very aggressive.*

Although Debbie expressed how such an unstructured and 'ordinary' household could lend itself to facilitate people getting 'stuck', the paradox for Debbie was that this 'structure' gave her the impetus to move on in her life.

BS: So you were saying, it might have been an overload of therapy?

Debbie: *Yeah I think I do. I think I felt like that, but then that might have been my resistance, but I don't know. I felt some people might have found it quite hard to find something else to fill the gaps where all the therapy was and they did not really help me with that. I was lucky in a way because I did ... I never wanted to stay in it all. I could see beyond it all, whereas some people in the house had no idea what they wanted. At the end of it they kind of got stuck in the therapy, but that's my opinion. I could be completely wrong but I think that's partly why they did not want me to do the course because I was very conscious that I did not want to get stuck in it and that's why I wanted to do an educational course so I had something to move onto.*

BS: So you were doing the course and you wanted a life to move onto after it.

Debbie: *Yeah. I wanted a way out and I think I always knew that it was not going to be something I would do for the rest of my life. So it was a way of getting out and it was. I nearly did something else, I needed something else to hide behind when I left because I could just say I am a lone female and I do it. Yeah, I don't think I would have had the confidence to just go for a job, because I had not worked for over eight years or whatever. Then people would ask questions ... that's how I did it. I don't know how other people do it. There are different ways.*

BS: What did you think was helpful and unhelpful about your experience in the house?

Debbie: *Helpful things were like, you could stay there as long as you liked, they did not throw you out, living with other people, having the house meetings, having the therapists always there. Really they were always brilliant whether you liked them or not at the time. They were always there. I guess the freedom ... you had a certain freedom as well as the rules of the house. You had a lot of freedom to do anything else you wanted really. The people most of the time. I mean you never get to stay (X) years in other places* [in reference to the length of time she stayed in the PA community house]. *I guess it was a home. It wasn't just a hostel or whatever. It was a home. It was never meant to be a short-stay place. It was meant to be somewhere where you made your home. That was very positive. They always encouraged you to feel at home, do what you want in your home.*

Unhelpful [things in the PA house]: *I think was the amount of therapy, but again I don't know if that was unhelpful at all. I think it just felt unhelpful at the time but that might have just been because you wanted to do something else instead of doing therapy every day all the time. I can't really think of unhelpful things. I mean I know a lot of the time you want to leave and stuff, but I don't think that would have been helpful. I can't really think of any unhelpful things. Maybe things like leaving was very difficult, but I don't think it could have been made any easier.*

Debbie described quite beautifully how she managed the awkward dilemma of many people suffering from mental distress, of having to get on and do things; this idea of doing things is rife in most areas of mental health care. Debbie's solution to this was again, what would seem to many action-orientated mental health professionals, unthinkable.[1]

BS: When you first moved into the houses you said you wanted somewhere to stay and help. So you had those wishes of help and that's what you wanted to get out of it. So I suppose the question is (1) do you feel you got that? and (2) is there anything you felt you did not get?

Debbie: *Well, I don't know, it's always easier to say in hindsight isn't it because I am happy I can't think of anything else I would rather have apart from what I have. So none of it has been easy. I don't think you ever leave and I think your life is fine. I mean I definitely felt I had been helped without a doubt, but I mean years after leaving it was still difficult and I had difficult times. I think you learn when you are in the house when you are having difficult times they pass, things change and get better, even if you just sit still you sort of have this attitude that when things are really awful I would just sit still and just wait and time would pass, then I would go to bed and the next day I would be better or I don't know, things always changed. I just learned that in the house, if you did not run away it would still get better, even if you did nothing. I think the house therapists were into this thing you know* [the positivity of not running away from mental distress and staying with it]. *People often think they have to do something to change, however actually I think I learned how not to do anything and that things would change and that they would change by themselves. I don't know what I am on about (laughs).*

BS: No, no, it sounds very interesting.

Debbie: *Yeah, but I think that has really helped me over the years, not to panic if you are feeling bad, not to fear the end of the world, not to feel you have to change something about your life or you have to do something. Sometimes you do have to do something, but you don't have to do them in the moment, just wait until you feel a bit better so then do something rather than trying to do something at the time when you are feeling really bad. So yes one of the things we learned was to tolerate things when we were really bad without trying to make it go away. That is something very important that I learned in the house; just tolerate my own feelings of badness and not try to make them go away. And yeah, they pass on their own, and when that happens over and over again even when you have left the house you just think, oh well, I'll just have to wait for this to pass and when you feel better you can try again.*

BS: It sounds very much like a kind of paradoxical kind of reality or way to get 'better'?

Debbie: *Yeah …*

BS: … From maybe a more proactive way of dealing with mental health problems, getting things done and doing things?

Debbie: *Yeah. To bear it, and if you can bear it then you are not frightened of it and I used to feel so frightened of feeling so bad I could not stand it. Then you think, oh well, I have been through it before, I can go through it again, the more times you go through it, the less bad it is or the less frightened you are. So I guess you learn that and that helps with the time. The fact that you are in the house for such a long time helps you go through it enough times that you do begin to feel more confident … I guess to do it on your own. I don't think there is an easy solution. It is not a miracle cure, you still have to do a lot of work even when you leave the house, that is how it happens, just by experiencing it, you learn from your experiences, and then you have those experiences and that's how you carry on.*

BS: It sounds like a constant coming up against your fears instead of retreating away which could be accomplished I suppose through the use of drugs for example, which might suppress distress?

Debbie: *Yeah, just because you're in the house and you can't run away, that's how it works, I don't know what you would call it. Maybe intense things like phobias, you have to face your phobia over and over again and it diminishes I guess.*

BS: What are your last thoughts and reflections about the house since you left the house?

Debbie: *I suppose now is the time now I feel I can relax. It is like a constant mountain to climb, nothing has been easy, but I suppose I have had an idea of what I wanted and also it's about fitting in to normal life. When you have been ill for a long time, I was ill for a long time before I went into the house, then I was in the house for (X amount of) years, you are kind of in this other world really which is quite different from normal life. I feel more adjusted to life than I have ever done, but nobody would ever know that I had any problems, I don't know if that is a good thing or a bad thing. I suppose it is a good thing. I guess I feel more confident with people. Yeah, nobody exists that does not have problems. You kind of learn that everybody has their things, that they worry about things, that they struggle with things like everybody else. These* [Debbie points to her children] *have kept me busy for years ... that's not been easy. It's just the capacity to learn, if you have not got that ... if someone has helped you to learn that, to learn from life, to cope with the knocks and scrapes and things like that then you can carry on.*

BS: It sounds like a very ordinary kind of way of working through things?

Debbie: *It's very ordinary. My life is the most ordinary life you can ever imagine, but that's all I ever wanted. Some people might want something fantastic from life, but you know, I don't think I knew that originally, as it turns out it's pretty good.*

BS: I did not mean that your life was very ordinary but that the whole kind of process is quite an ordinary kind of process ... there does not seem to be anything fancy in the process you described?

Debbie: *No, I don't think there is. You know, the humdrum, accepting the humdrumness of life, that's what it's about. For me, I have worked god knows how many years to get to this point, so for some people they would think that this is just ordinary life, this is not any achievement or anything, it just happens to them. Like my friends think, this is how everyone's life is. They don't think twice about it, but I am very conscious that it is an achievement and I think it probably makes me happier a lot of the time. Happier because I get moments where I think ... wow ... isn't this great! I am really lucky. Maybe other people don't think how lucky they are. In some ways it's easier to appreciate the simpler things. I don't take things for granted. It's just life isn't it? It's hard to put it all into context sometimes, the whole PA experience, especially as the years pass. It's almost becomes a dream; did it ever happen, who are (the house therapists)? I mean we have our Christmas exchange of emails. Sometimes that feels difficult but it also feels nice that I still have that contact with them. Sometimes that feels very strange. It's not like leaving home where you can go back, have Sunday lunch, take your washing back, it's not like that. You never see them again. I do know that is how it is. But it's still bad. There is still a bit of badness around it. But you have to be like that. But I am lucky that it does not bother me too much. I have got things to keep me busy but again I can imagine this is something that I imagine some people find difficult; leaving and no contact. But there is not any better way of doing it. You can't have people hanging around and coming to meetings and I have been back a few times for events etc.*

Endnote

1. 'Action-orientated mental health professional' implies somebody frantically searching and grasping to cure their patients, to treat their patients, to alleviate their suffering.

Chapter Eighteen

Lyn

Lyn was inspired to come to the PA after reading some of the works of R.D. Laing. She found a resonance with his material and her own life. Lyn was also suffering from much depression and her call to the PA was very much influenced by her distress, although this was not wholly apparent at the time of her move into the PA community.

Lyn: *I was (X) years old and I had read* The Politics of Experience *and whatever it was* [or another book by R.D. Laing]. *I had nothing to do with therapy, I had no idea … but I had read* The Politics of Experience *and I can remember reading that, I can remember the day and I just read it cover to cover … and I just wept and wept because I thought, oh my God, this experience I had with my family, obviously I was not the only one … there is a language for it* [her distress and her experience] *and for me it … I was a kind of budding socialist I think at the time, so for me it was all about politics, that's why I picked up the book. I didn't read* The Divided Self [another book by R.D. Laing] *first, I read* Politics of Experience *… We* [Lyn's partner at the time] *were going to come to Europe … and we were going to end up in London for a few months. So I thought God, I've got to find this guy, who is this R.D. Laing? It was like you know, how you talked about the light* [of the PA][1] *… I did not know it at the time, but I was depressed and I had a lot of angst.*

Having grown up in a crappy middle-class family and you know, double-binded [by her family], *so I just wanted to meet him. Where I came from there was no concept of therapy. People went to psychiatrists who were in the mental hospital. Before the 1970s people didn't go into therapy, well not where I came from … I showed up here at the PA because I had this inexplicable sadness and 'lost-ness'. I had been considering suicide for a couple of years. I wasn't taking any drugs, some but not enough to really push me over the edge. I realise after being here* [in London with the PA] *that it was really quite a blessing that my parents didn't really know that I was depressed; everybody else that ends up like that ends up in a mental hospital.*

My way of coping in life was to take care of people ... I kind of thought I am here to help others so I am going to go into the [PA] *houses to help people which of course I learned very quickly help was a terribly dirty word* [in the PA houses]; *'Who do you think you are that you can help anybody?'* [was the kind of response she encountered].

As a result of this experience of going into the house thinking she was going to 'help people' and being confronted with her own motives and depression, the journey of trying to get to grips with herself began. She began to realise that the house was very much a saviour for her.

Lyn: *I had a really hard time trying to define myself as helper or a depressed person. I realised later and at the time as well that my life depended on being in the house. I look back on it and think I probably would have ended up in a psychiatric hospital like a lot of my friends did in those days ... having the validation was incredibly important that whatever I was experiencing was real, having the camaraderie and for me the intellectual stimulation, the incredible rigour of it all.*

The blurring of boundaries between residents, therapists and live-in trainee therapists who were training in the PA was something quite apparent in the PA house that Lyn lived in.[2]

Lyn: *There was no staff, everybody was all in it together, except whoever the house therapist was, who were paid to come around to the house. But anybody else there who had any illusions that they were an intern* [trainee therapist] *or anything else were shredded constantly. You know, it was a 'you are just one of us' kind of thing. And it* [this blurring of boundaries] *was true and that's what kept me there because of the authenticity of it all.*

Lyn went on to discuss the criticism (some people's) that R.D. Laing glorified and romanticised madness with his PA houses experiments.

However, Lyn had a different take on this, that the PA communities should be on the 'edge', subversive, and delineated from conventional psychiatric and psychotherapeutic treatment to enable the PA communities to grow and survive.

Lyn: *I could talk for hours what I learned from my experience in the PA. In order to change anything, you do have to glorify whatever it is for a while; you have to take it to this extreme. I think that the thing about the PA is that it was an experiment and that it has to stay out on the edge, push the envelope and the envelope was being pushed at the time in regards what was going on politically. Anti-psychiatry was the thing of the day, but yes, I have talked to people about being in a PA house … this is my opinion, the diagnosis of schizophrenia and schizoid personality disorders, there is a whole range of people who are misdiagnosed. I think there are some people for whom those diagnoses seem to fit a bit and within those people there are people who do very well in a structured environment and people who don't. What you find out is that even if you subscribe to some theory that there are some people who are psychotic and they are different from you and me, suppose you subscribe to that, they are not all that different and at the bottom of it it's all understandable* [people in mental distress]. *This is the gift I got from being in the PA house, being in it, being on the edge of my own madness, which in my case was depression.*

Lyn describes the importance of being in the environment of the PA houses where 'us and them' definitions, psychiatric diagnosis, and labels were not considered important, but having to be 'there' for other people was. This dynamic was one of the facets of her experience in the house which helped her own mental distress. Lyn describes this beautifully.

Lyn: *So the other thing that I really learned from being in the PA house was that the path out of depression is service to others. I really got that and that served me over the years. Yeah, I was really depressed and suicidal but this woman over here or this woman over there* [in the house], *they were literally fighting with the devil for their life in that moment. And I said to myself, OK, I can come out of my depression for a moment and then help in a way that wasn't ego-based; it was being with them, and they were with me. It was quite amazing.*

Later in the conversation I described my own experience with 'depression' and my own experience in psychotherapy. This struck a chord with Lyn in her understanding of how we can 'get out' of our 'depressions'.

BS: I would go in to see my therapist and say something like that I was depressed or whatever and he would just laugh at me. You know he would not actually do anything. I mean therapy can be quite a narcissistic thing, depression can be quite narcissistic and some people ask me what my therapy was like and I sometimes reply that it's kind of like a weird kind of shamanic thing … you go into a room to meet somebody and they don't actually do anything, but you come out feeling better. I say to myself after such experiences, how the hell do I feel better? Nothing has been done [to me]. Maybe my therapist has even talked about himself for the 50 minutes and it's like a completely different human being that I have become. So how the hell do you regulate that?[3] Do you see where I am coming from?

(Both laugh)

Lyn: *Absolutely. Actually it's funny that you should bring up that word 'shamanism'. One of the things that really impacted on me was reading Francis Huxley*[4] *… Huxley was this anthropologist who talked to us about shamans walking between two worlds and I had. I grew up on an Indian reservation. My father worked for the government and I had quite a few pretty amazing experiences as a child that I took for granted. I never really thought much about them until much later …*

Lyn has read widely and developed a keen interest (which she still has) in alternative healing methods along with traditional psychotherapy. She described some of this during our conversation and how she felt that such 'practices' were part of the PA house experience.

Lyn: *I got much more into Jung … and the shamanic world with psychoanalysis, phenomenology and so forth, particularly all this kind of Maurice Merleau-Ponty stuff that I read. I then got into the body and embodiment, the world of the imaginal and how one could use guided imagery to move through real life experiences ... if we do guided imagery and you have an imaginal experience the body reacts to it as though it actually experienced it, which is shamanism ... The shamanism that was flying around here* [the PA House] *consciously and unconsciously ... Ronnie* [Laing] *was certainly a shaman. I mean the shaman walks between two worlds ... the daily experience of ego-shattering living in the house and having one's assumptions and one's being challenged is again shamanic. That is the truth about what shamans are* [what they do: shattering one's ego] *... once a year they* [shamans] *stand there and yank out their own hearts and let the vultures eat it so they can be reborn and that's what was going on in the PA house ... you had to walk between two worlds to survive ... and when you have had these experiences ... you've got it ... what they say about the shamans is that you have to go through things like that* [personal suffering and illness]. *I think that's what things like depression are; it is a shamanic initiation.*

The idea of love was brought by Lyn as an important aspect of the experience of being in a PA household. This was mixed in with the idea that the experience of being in the house and going through her depression there was invaluable for her when she experienced depression after she left the house.

Lyn: *... so that's a kind of a long way round of my experience which really started with suicidal depression which I feel was treated and cured in a PA household. It gave me a foundation so that when I did have a major depressive episode later, I didn't think that I had to go to hospital. I understood what it meant and I think that must be true ... I think that the people that were there were loved, supported, had incredible insight, had conversion experiences, which they would never have had if they had been drugged up and in a psychiatric hospital ... one thing I have is this visceral memory of the feeling of waking up* [in a PA house] *and thinking, what will be happening today? Because it was not predictable and I think that unpredictability was the authenticity and you would get up in the morning and come downstairs; there might be nobody there, it might be empty or there might already be people down there smoking cigarettes ...*

... and there would be business of how are we going to get through the day. I mean one of the residents was lying upstairs in bed and had not got out of his bed for ages; somebody has got to sit with him. So the one thing about it was a

lot of communication had to happen and it had to be authentic communication ... other than that there was the ordinary business of living your life was what was important.

Like for many who have lived in the PA houses, the difficulties were plainly evident, and again the quest for authenticity perhaps contributed to this, but paradoxically this seems to be one reason why Lyn feels she benefited from the house, as a result of the compassion that it engendered.

Lyn: *There was a lot of bickering because we were all there projecting onto each other; all of our family of origin issues. So the house was filled with ghosts of my own and other people's mums, fathers, sisters, brothers and everybody else, and everybody that reminded me of them or didn't remind me of them. It was absolute madness. Honestly, what held it all together was the quest for authenticity and there was this ... I think it was a good experiment in ontological compassion as well ... there was no reason we had to be nice to each other, but the kind of Lord-of-the-Flies kind of environment, the who is going to rule today? ... I mean who had the greatest need to be the leader ... I had a lot of control issues. I wanted to fix everything all the time. My father was an alcoholic, my mother was severely depressed. My sister had a physical handicap. So I came with all that baggage and I wanted to help everybody and others loved to be helped. But then of course what really held it together was the house therapist coming round three or four times a week ...*

... then often there was this sense of safety in just being in the house and that the world out there was a little bit of a scary place. It was a cocooned feeling and by safe I mean it was a place where you could be authentic, where you were going to have a real connection with people. People were quite protective toward each other for the most part ... the love and compassion in the household was tremendous [from residents and therapists] *... what was terrifying was that I knew I would be seen, that my own shadow would be called out. It really scared me. I just felt like I was like this little girl ... that I didn't know anything and I was naïve and arrogant ... I was afraid of being seen. I rarely was ever afraid of physical stuff; that was very rare. I was afraid of being found out, not being good enough. I was worried by these people I was living with in the house that seemed to be plugged into something ... and as Laing would say, and they were, they*

really were shamans themselves. And it is sad for them that they [some therapists and residents] *that they were often stuck in that role and getting hurt for it. Yeah, I had to learn to communicate authentically at a very young age and to be sensitive in that environment.*

But it was not all seriousness in the PA house. Lyn described another more humorous side of the experience of living in the house.

Lyn: *We had lots of fun, that's the other thing. There were lots of laughs all through the PA; a sense of humour, the sardonic, the absurdity of life, the cosmic joke or whatnot was about all the time.*

The topic of love was mentioned several times during our conversation and I wanted to know more about this as other people I had interviewed had mentioned this.

BS: A few other people I have interviewed have mentioned love in their interviews. They said that the therapists loved us. It is an amazing thing to hear that. When I was doing my training [psychotherapy training at the Philadelphia Association], and I don't mean to go on about it, but maybe it's helpful.

Lyn: *It's very helpful.*

BS: When I was doing my training I told my supervisor at the time, James Low, he has studied Buddhism, so he is into that sort of stuff ... and I said to him, this job as a therapist ... it struck me the other day when I was sitting with a patient, and it actually struck me also as a result of an experience I had with my wife ... you know, you are sitting opposite a person, another human being, and you look at them, and a sudden realisation came over me, which has happened with patients and in other contexts with people, and I thought, oh my God, the fragility of this other person, it's actually quite painful to see it. And you know what I am getting at ... to revert to a more ego-bound way of functioning kind of protects you from this painful realisation [of the fragility of the Other].

Lyn: *Exactly, you're right, your whole heart ... people who work in psychiatric hospitals, that I think are objectifying, they are just scared and what they are afraid of is their own heartache, their own fragility. They really have those experiences you're describing. You said it beautifully.*

... So that fragility and when you keep your heart open it's painful. That's what shamans are talking about. They pull their heart out and let the vultures pick at it. That's how you stay alive. There is a Leon Redler [a PA therapist] *story that I heard him tell. There is a Buddhist saying, when you have an open heart, you can see your spine. So in other words that's your strength as opposed to ego. The fact that an open heart makes you weak or vulnerable, it doesn't. I think that's what we got* [learned in the house] *as opposed to ordinary psychiatric or psychological experiences* [objectifying ideas about mental health]. *We learned that an open heart is what makes it possible. What else was I going to do but open my heart? Well I got stabbed a few times, metaphorically speaking, and then you learn over the years to open it up. It's easier than not doing so.*

The conversation continued on this topic, talking about the heart and fragility of people. I described to Lyn an experience or practice where one just sits opposite somebody and stares at their eyes for a prolonged period of time: 5–10 minutes or more.

BS: I carried this out at a conference in Switzerland with a Dutchman who I met and subsequently became friends with. It was a powerful experience that was 'ego-breaking' but also made me feel very open and compassionate with this fellow I met. It was a very powerful experience which I feel facilitated an openness and pulled down the barriers of what Levinas might call the totalisation of the other.

Lyn: *It seems that what you are talking about is I think what we started with talking about. Here's the connection; living in the household, those kinds of experiences went on. There were people sitting across from each other, gazing into each other's eyes, people staying up all night together looking into the fire. And as you experienced, this can create the kind of authenticity that occurred in the households ... but they are real experiences. You didn't know this Dutch guy and think about how quick that took to feel that compassion; 5–10 minutes?*

BS: Yes.

Lyn: *I think those things* [the 'staring/being with another' experiences we were discussing] *are as potent, more potent than talking therapy. When you combine them with talk therapy, when you combine the experiential moment, like that, and there are lots of other experiences, they create this authentic space, and then to interpret and then to do talk therapy. So I know exactly what you are talking about. Part of it is just taking time to be together. I mean, just look what we are doing, we have a reason to be together today, and I feel I kind of know you today.*

BS: Yes, yes, I agree.

Lyn: *You know a very real connection, that capacity that we are having to feel this with each other, to get to know you better ... that's got to be therapeutic. It is got to be what it is about, and that's love.*

BS: Yes!

Lyn: *That's just loving who you are and who you are with. Do you know the term 'Namaste'* [a Sanskrit term] *and what it means? It means I bow to the God within you. It's your soul you know ... we are bowing to each other's soul.*

BS: It's deep and profound stuff isn't it!

Lyn: *Amazing stuff ...*

Endnotes

1. I had mentioned to Lyn before we started recording that I saw the PA in terms of being a beacon of light in a dark world; the PA is 'en-lightened' (or can be) by its critical stance towards the 'dark' (uncritical of dogma) medical and scientific accounts of mental distress.
2. Lyn's period in the houses was when there was a very blurred distinction between different kinds of residents; trainee therapists, patients, therapists, and other interested parties.

3. The reference to regulation is in the context of the push for regulation by the Health and Care Professions Council (HCPC) in the UK. We discussed this in conversation before recording began. At the time of this recording (2010) the HCPC (then known as the Health Professions Council) wanted to regulate the minutiae of the therapeutic encounter between therapist and patient. This is outlined in the Maresfield Report (http://www.psychoanalysis-cpuk.org/HTML/RegulationArchive/Reports.htm), a document published as a challenge to the proposals of setting standards of therapeutic practice by the HCPC. The Philadelphia Association was one of the psychoanalytic groups involved with this publication.
4. Francis Huxley was involved with the PA and the PA communities during the 1970s. He has written widely on the topics of psychoanalysis, anthropology, and shamanism.

Part 3

Tales of *Docta Ignorantia*: Analysis of interviews

Chapter Nineteen

The unveiling and re-veiling of a research schema and *Docta Ignorantia*: Approaching an analysis of the interviews

Introduction to *Docta Ignorantia*

I am with Feyerabend (1975) and his idea of proceeding counter-intuitively (against the logical-positivist position), to be very wary of building a system or taxonomy (qualitative or quantitative) of what works and what does not work in the healing of people who live in a Philadelphia Association community house. I am proposing to *out* a paradox, or at the very least unveil the paradox for an instant, if such a thing is possible. No doubt, upon analysing the interviews with all the verve of a qualitative researcher, trying to find themes, codes, systems and taxonomies, I could have devised a structure or structures that depicted the ideal route to healing mental distress for people who have lived in these communities, but unfortunately, paradox, contradiction, rabbit holes, dead ends, and chasing my own tail reared their heads time and time again.[1] This perplexity perplexed me, but I realised that there might be honesty in this perplexity, beyond my logical reasoning powers. I believe I stumbled upon the *Docta Ignorantia,* or the doctrine of learned or wise ignorance, in my research journey. *Docta Ignorantia* was a term coined by Nicolaus Cusanus, a fifteenth-century theologian and philosopher (Cusanus, 2007).

Docta Ignorantia has its origins in the ideas of Parmenides, followed by Plato, and today traces of it remain in the likes of Kierkegaard, Wittgenstein, Derrida, and the psychoanalyst Jacques Lacan. Cusanus, like Parmenides, shows how 'finite' thought is limited and betrays our fundamental capacities of (or *for*) not-knowing and the infinitude of *Being* that constantly get sidelined when we place finitude upon the world via our scientistic posturing. We close off the possibility of the text, as Derrida (1997) might say. Cusanus demonstrated our fundamental wrong-turning of relying upon human intellect by showing through the examples of comparing and contrasting finite and infinite lines, circles and triangles, how our limited human conceptualisation and cogitation can only reveal to a certain point. Montaigne (1991) takes up this point in his essays showing how we have to err on the path of life to uncover what we cannot uncover through a rational intellectual process. Thus, as Heidegger (2001) would attest, life unveils itself to us; we do not unveil life to ourselves, however hard we might try. However, as Hadot (2006) eloquently points out, as soon as life or nature unveils itself, it becomes veiled again – a situation that can never be manipulated (by our will) where nature or human living becomes permanently unveiled and known to cogitation and reason. Hadot's analysis, I believe, was reflected in the diachrony, or the lack of synchrony, within the interviews of ex-residents: *Docta Ignorantia*.

Analysis of interviews: Approaching *Docta Ignorantia*

The analysis of the interviews did not take the usual qualitative path as used within university discourse – i.e., creating universal truths or applicable theory to a collective (see Lacan, 2007, regarding his critique of the university discourse). There were reasons for this.

The first reason, as already discussed in Chapter 3, was that no proposed theory building was actively sought; this would have been contrary to the activity of what occurs in the houses. In other words, a predestined journey (based on a theory) for a resident within the household would have been contra-indicative of that journey or experience to be experienced. The house therapists neither impose a treatment plan on residents nor have preconceived ideas of how a resident should 'progress'. (See Gordon, 2010, for a wonderful and informative description of the Philadelphia Association communities.) Therefore if you introduce a theory to be taken and used by others it introduces a component which would not be what one sought or wished to introduce. In other words, one would have the situation of Baudrillard's (1994) simulacra and simulation; one would have a replica of a hypothesised model intruding upon the scene of another context. This is, in effect, to use scientific jargon, contamination of the scientific field.

The second reason, leading on from the first, is based upon the psycho-scientific fallacy. This is the fallacy of obtaining objective facts, generalisable facts that can form a model or theory that can be applied in other contexts within the (loosely speaking) psychological sphere. The problem with this approach is that any validity or reliability is nullified as replication becomes a meaningless, ungraspable, and infinite exercise (Feyerabend, 1975). This is because what occurs (or at least is attempted, but not always completely successfully) in the Philadelphia Association community households is nothing more mysterious than trying to let other people be and find their own voice and health in their own time:

autorhythmia. Each story and each individual are different. Therefore to generalise research 'findings' to other people and contexts as if this is *the formula* would be a very precarious business and an obtuse procedure leading to mystifications and confusions. From a scientific point of view such generalisations would be meaningless. In the present study, to comply with empirical-logistic-scientific methodology, as discussed in Chapter 3, one would have to take into account so many variables that it would be impossible for replication in a subsequent study; providing a scientific account would be very unscientific. Of course, there may be aspects of the praxis of living in a PA house that can be ascertained and deliberated on, but ultimately, each individual has to find their own individual healing praxis; that includes therapist, researcher, and resident of a community household. In other words, something or some phenomena may emerge on the micro level of an individual and the macro level of the group. But let us go further: something may be operating in 'healing' that is beyond pinpointing agency and rationalisation (on the micro and macro level) and more importantly, as soon as we rationalise this process, or rather praxis, it is lost; dogmatic posturing has no place in the solution to human suffering as Kierkegaard would attest (Kierkegaard, 1975).

This takes me now to the place where I do indeed rely upon a schema (or structure of kinds, but perhaps a *de-con-structure*), which led me to identify the appearance of *Docta Ignorantia* in my methodology and how I analysed the results of my research. However, I believe this schema shows not a method, but rather an anti-method which unveils un-knowing – an un-knowing that embodies the erring way depicted by Cusanus (2007), Montaigne (1991), Kierkegaard (1975), Plato (in Cooper, 1997), Parmenides (in Geldard, 2007), and Derrida (1997); this leads to a wise ignorance, or as Kierkegaard (1975) might say, the paradox of reason leading to freedom from the tyranny of cogitation and systemisation. In analysing the interviews of the ex-residents of the PA community houses I indeed came upon paradox, where system building failed me. See Figure 1 (overleaf).

This schema outlines the discourses I identified in the interviewees' transcripts and how they are constructed or built up in stages 1–4. These are fluid and interchangeable discourses; the discourses are not fixed states or even meant to represent a hierarchical statement or schema or process. All interviewees could have possibly gone through all eight discourses of stage 4 (A.–H) at some point in their life trajectory, as we all can experience at some point. Some interviewees showed more dominant discourses from stage 4 (e.g., E or F) or went through periods of interchanging discourses. They represent not so much a process, but a praxis which eludes pinning a process onto it that subsequently can be controlled from outside.

Figure 1: Schema of interviewees' discourse

1. Interviewees' experience

2. Knowing or Not-Knowing (the problem, their mental distress, and thinking they can fix it/cure themselves)

A – Knowing or thinking they can fix or cure themselves

B – Not-Knowing or thinking they cannot fix or cure themselves

3. Knower's and Not-Knower's experiencing perplexity or experiencing calm in relation to their state of mental distress

A – Knower + Calm // **B** – Knower + Perplexity

C – Not-Knower + Calm // **D** – Not-Knower + Perplexity

4. Knower's and Not-Knower's (how to fix their mental distress) experiencing calm or perplexity in relation to mental distress, and either grasping after a cure or not grasping after a cure (i.e., dwelling in negative capability[2])

A – Knower + Calm + Grasping // **B** – Knower + Calm + Negative Capability

C – Knower + Perplexity + Grasping // **D** – Knower + Perplexity + Negative Capability

E – Not-Knower + Calm + Grasping // **F** – Not-Knower + Calm + Negative Capability

G – Not-Knower + Perplexity + Grasping // **H** – Not-Knower + Perplexity + Negative Capability

What was remarkable was that applying Lacan's four-discourse theory (Lacan, 2007, see Figures 2 and 3 below) separated the interviewees' discourses into three types from stage 4: one type in comprising discourses A, C, E and G, a second type in discourses B and D, and a third type in discourses F and H. However, discourses B, D, F and H are related in a paradoxical way as I will describe below.

Firstly however, a few words on Lacan's discourse theory are needed before we proceed. It can be stated that Lacan's ideas on discourse point to a *Docta Ignorantia* that epitomises the human condition or human communication. His theory is in radical opposition to communication theory for example (i.e., perfect information transfer). In other words Lacan starts from the assumption that communication between people is always a failure; it has to be a failure because this is the reason we continue to speak to one another. If we communicated perfectly to each other we would remain silent. The discourses reflect this impossibility of Truth with a capital T, Knowledge with a capital K, and the realisation of the impossibility of a unified subject – a *Docta Ignorantia* (Lacan, 2007).

As you can see from Figure 2 below, the structure of the discourses comprises four positions and two disjunctions. These four positions of agent, other, product, and truth (which I will explain below), and the two disjunctions (which are interrelated) show the disruption of the lines of communication between people.

The disjunction of impossibility (symbolised with an arrow pointing right on the upper level) rests with the agent. The agent (with complete knowing volition) is a fiction. The agent is driven by a desire which constitutes their truth. The truth cannot be completely verbalised, with the result that the agent cannot transmit his or her desire to the other. Therefore a perfect communication with words is logically impossible. Lacan (2007) goes much further in his discussion regarding this, but sufficient for our purposes here, the bridge between the agent and other is always a bridge too far, with the result that the agent remains fixed with an impossible desire. Therefore, each of the four discourses (see Figure 3) unites a group of subjects through a particular impossibility of a particular desire.

On the lower level of the discourse theory (see Figure 2) we have the disjunction of inability symbolised with //. This inability concerns the link between product and truth. The product, as a result of the discourse of the other, has nothing to do with the truth of the agent. If it was possible for an agent to verbalise the complete truth to the other, the other would respond with an appropriate product. However, as it is impossible to fulfil this condition, the product can never mirror what forms the basis of truth in the position of truth.

A further reason for the impossibility of human communication is as a result of the position of truth (left-hand bottom of Figure 2). It fuels the agent, but the agent is unaware of this truth; the agent is only apparently the agent. The ego does not speak, it is spoken. In other words, I do not speak, but I am spoken, and this speech is driven by a desire, with or without my conscious agreement. This is a matter of simple observation, but it is fundamentally wounding to man's narcissism. This echoes Kierkegaard's (1975) idea of the paradox of reason as discussed in Chapter 2.

Figure 2: Four positions

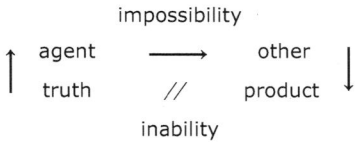

S_1, S_2, $, and objet petit a ($a$) rotate around the four positions (see Figure 3). You need at the very least two signifiers in order to have a minimal linguistic structure. S_1 is the first signifier, the Freudian border signifier, primary symbol, or primary symptom. It is the master-signifier, trying to fill up the lack (e.g., impossible desire, impossible communication), posturing as the guarantee for the process of covering up that lack. A good example is the signifier 'I' which gives us the illusion of an identity of our own. S_2 is the denominator for the rest of the signifiers, the chain or network of signifiers. In that sense, it is also the denominator of '*le savoir*', the knowledge which is contained in that chain of signifiers that are the foundation of a given discourse. This knowledge is not knowledge with a capital K or truth with a capital T; there is a lack within it as perfect communication is impossible and there is an inability to get to the position of truth.

The next two terms ($ and objet petit a) are both an effect of the signifier. Where we have two signifiers, the necessary condition for the existence of a subject is fulfilled (i.e., S_1 and S_2); a signifier is what represents a subject for another signifier. But as discussed above, communication is imperfect and the result is a divided subject ($). The final term is the lost objet petit a (a). The result of language acquisition is a loss of a primary condition, or being split off from nature. From the moment you speak, you become a subject of language, a divided subject who attempts to grasp an object beyond language, or, more precisely, a condition beyond the separation between subject and object. This object represents desire itself; it lies beyond the sphere of the signifier and consequently beyond the pleasure principle; it is irretrievably lost. It constitutes the engine that keeps humans desiring. As Lacan (2007) argued, it constitutes the basis of every form of causality for human experience.

This detour into Lacanian discourse theory informing my schema of the interviewees' discourses sheds light upon and lends weight to the concept of the impossibility of Knowing (with a capital K) Truth (with a capital T), and the impossibility of a unified subject. Discourses A, C, E and G could be subsumed, roughly speaking, under Lacan's discourse of

Figure 3: Four discourses

Four terms: Master signifier (S_1), knowledge (S_2), objet petit a (*a*), divided subject ($).

Discourse of the University

$$\uparrow \frac{S_2 \longrightarrow a}{S_1 \; // \; \$} \downarrow$$

Discourse of the Master

$$\uparrow \frac{S_1 \longrightarrow S_2}{\$ \; // \; a} \downarrow$$

Discourse of the Hysteric

$$\uparrow \frac{\$ \longrightarrow S_1}{a \; // \; S_2} \downarrow$$

Discourse of the Analyst

$$\uparrow \frac{a \longrightarrow \$}{S_2 \; // \; S_1} \downarrow$$

the master, the hysteric, or even the university. Discourses A and C from my schema are mostly similar to Lacan's discourse of the master. From the position of the agent (S_1 in the discourse of the master, the interviewee, as agent, believes he or she comes from a position of truth (they know or think that they can cure their mental distress and are grasping for a cure) and can get this cure or at least demand it from the other (S_2: psychiatrists, house therapists). But the agent in this position does not know he or she comes from a position of the barred (divided) subject ($), and is left with a product/lack which cannot satisfy desire (i.e., *a*). Kierkegaard's (1975) idea of the paradox of reason, where we cannot know all through cogitation in order to become happy/cured or get happiness, is reflected in this discourse. If a person is in the place of the *other* (S_2) in Lacan's discourse of the master, for example, taking orders from the psychiatric masters, or believing the house therapists are masters (S_1), they will know what they need to do when taking orders or knowledge from the masters, but they will not know why they do so. Thus, they will not know why/what they are producing (e.g progress, happiness etc.) and crucially they are still left bereft with lost object (*a*), and the resulting lack. The difference between my discourse A and C in which I link to Lacan's discourse of the master is the presence of perplexity and calmness: discourse A having calm and discourse C having perplexity. This makes the agent (with perplexity), in the position of S_1 in Lacan's discourse of the master as being a bit of a hysterical master, not sure of their position of master and what effect they will have on the other (S_2).

Discourses E and G of my schema are more similar to Lacan's discourse of the hysteric. A person in E and G in the position of the agent ($) in Lacan's discourse of the hysteric is in a position of a divided subject, not having ultimate truth or knowledge, but desiring, unawares, ultimate truth and knowledge (fuelled by position of truth and impossible desire and lack, *a*), and who demands from the other (S_1) knowledge in order to understand their way out of mental distress (e.g., asking psychiatrists or house therapists for the cure to mental distress in order to become an undivided subject). Unfortunately, this discourse does not bring ultimate truth, which the agent is grasping after; sure, the psychiatrist or house therapist might provide truth (S_2), but it will be a false truth as it will not be related specifically to their suffering, as it is a fictive truth (the person needs to find their own truthfulness, and also realise that the desire for ultimate Truth with a capital T is unobtainable), like the slave in Plato's dialogue *Meno* – see Plato, in Cooper, 1997, and the discussion, Chapter 21.

Or to put it in a different context, from the position of the other (S_1) in my discourses E and G, from Lacan's discourse of the hysteric, the other (interviewee or patient) will try to respond to the demands of the agent ($) (e.g., the demands of a therapist's/psychiatrist's discourse worrying about mentally ill people having to get better). Again this will produce only more knowledge, which will not be ultimate truth for the person as they have to find their own truth, or rather, their own path into truthfulness.

However, in my discourse E, the added dimension, calmness, could indicate some similarity with Lacan's discourse of the university. In E from the position of agent (S_2) in the discourse of the university, the agent may believe that he or she will provide information (for the psychiatrists or house therapists; the position of the other *a*) so that they will teach them and they (the psychiatrists or house therapists) will therefore learn from them (the agent) and thus be able to cure them (the agent) but (paradoxically) reverting the agent back to the position of the other (S_2) as in the discourse of the master, or the position of agent ($) in the discourse of the hysteric. Alternatively, from the position of the other *a*, in the discourse of the university, the person may believe that he or she can learn (from the psychiatrists or house therapists). But from either position of agent, (S_2) or other (*a*) in the discourse of the university, ultimate truth is evaded; i.e., illusory ultimate truths/primary signifier (S_1) in the position of agent (S_2), drives the agent, and in the position of the other (S_2), the subject still remains divided by being fed or producing false truth of ultimate knowledge leading to a divided or barred subject ($).

Ultimately, the group of discourses in A, C, E and G belongs to a type of discourse where ultimate knowledge is desired or is thought to be obtainable (e.g., cure for mental distress). However, as Lacan (2007) pointed out, the discourses of the master, hysteric and university still leave the subject ultimately divided: they do not get their knowledge; it is an illusion; one can never really get 'it', as human ratiocination is finite, limited, and there are always other ideas or ways to know; living a human life, a good life in truthfulness, is something one has to find in one's own truthfulness, and it cannot be delivered like a formula (Derrida, 1997; Montaigne, 1991; Cusanus, 2007; Kierkegaard, 1975; Plato, in Cooper, 1997).

The discourses B and D seem to me to represent (in some ways and not in others) transition discourses from the discourse of A, C, E and G. In other words, with the addition of the quality of negative capability (not grasping after ultimate knowledge or the cure for mental distress), the need, desire, for ultimate truth with a capital T loses its hold, although there are still strains of the idea of ultimate knowledge or truth as depicted in Lacan's discourses of the master, hysteric and university; there is still some element of sureness of knowing or getting ultimate truth or curing mental distress (i.e., knowing the problem of mental distress and knowing/thinking one can cure it). However, with negative capability present in B and D, the drive for this truth becomes unimportant. Also in discourse D there is perplexity, but perplexity in itself is not serious; we can all experience perplexity and it is a necessity for overcoming our human suffering (and addiction to searching for ultimate truths regarding the human condition) as I will show and describe in the next chapter (see Almond, 2004, in his review of the philosophy of Ibn 'Arabi and Jacques Derrida, in relation to the necessity of perplexity in the human condition). However, the discourses of B and D hold similarities, paradoxically of not-knowing, which are related to the third set of discourses from my schema F and H; this is related to the idea of knowing that one does not know and being able to rest without grasping or desiring to cancel out the lack that is the human condition.

The third set of discourses (F and H) from my schema relate very well to Lacan's discourse of the analyst. In the discourse of the analyst, the agent (a) addresses the barred or divided subject ($\$$), which produces knowledge (S_1) that is not connected to the knowledge of the analyst. To put this in the perspective of my discourses F and H, the interviewee/ex-resident in the place of the other ($\$$) is left to create his or her own knowledge or truthfulness – not being told what is the truth via the discourse of the master or university, or being told to find the truth from the perspective of the discourse of the hysteric. But it does not stop here. As the agent remains in the place of unknowable desire (a), and even though the other ($\$$) is complicit in producing knowledge (S_1), the other ($\$$) still is left without ultimate knowledge or ultimate truth as the agent (a) is unknowable and thus it becomes an infinite task of circulating within this discourse. This is precisely why the practice of psychoanalysis or psychoanalytic-type work is a praxis and not a treatment with end goals as such. It is the infinite negotiation, awareness, and practice of impossibility within discourse and human communication. This is why such a practice is a *Docta Ignorantia*.

Being in the place of the agent in the discourse of the analyst, in the context of my discourses F and H, puts the agent (*a*) (interviewee/ex-resident) in a place where he or she lets the other barred or divided subject ($) (house therapist, other residents) create their own truth. In effect they do not lay anything on them or expect anything from them. This is in effect the Levinasian respect for the other, an act of non-totalisation (see Levinas, 1998, 2007). Of course by reaching the stage of F and H, one might arrive at a place where one knows that one does not know, which is a kind of knowing, and at the same time experience either calmness or perplexity.

My schema of the interviewees' discourse is not a static model, but I hope it shows the importance of negative capability and how this relates to *Docta Ignorantia* or wise unknowing as depicted in Lacan's (2007) discourse theory and his theory of psychoanalytic praxis. In each of these stages, because of the employment of negative capability, there is an appreciation and honouring of infinitely evolving and/or changing knowledge, or the realisation one can never get ultimate knowledge (in the place of the agent), and if in the place of the other, the opportunity to realise this. This discourse epitomises Aristotle's idea of praxis (see Heaton, 1998; Dunne, 1993; as discussed in Chapter 3), carrying out an activity for the sake of doing it, not for a product at the end of a process. One does end up with a product (some kind of knowledge in the discourse of the analyst or in my discourses B, D, F and H) but it is never finalised or cast in stone; one is forever doomed to be alienated from language and ultimate knowledge and be a divided subject. However, if one can tolerate this alienation or lack and employ negative capability, then one could possibly come to rest (not literally become stagnant, but able to respond to life) in a praxis of peacefulness.

My schema of the discourses that I identified in the interviewees' narratives and my linking of these to Lacan's four discourses theory is not meant to be a precise, perfect or definitive exposition of Lacanian theory to the results of the research, but a way of presenting the praxis of what goes on in the narratives: *Docta Ignorantia*, the paradox of reasoning, or the mess one can get into by searching after ultimate knowledge (in this case of finding the cure for mental distress). Ultimate knowledge, in the case of the experience of interviewees/ex-residents, or from the analysis of the interviews, was not and could not be forthcoming as there is no ultimate knowledge to be had in the ratiocination or reasoning for a cure for mental distress. What emerged as a theme from the interviews was that coming to one's own mind through such a praxis (finding peace, a way out of mental distress) involved a negative capability and wise unknowing (and a praxis of finding this and losing it and re-finding it and/or being patient in finding it/not finding it); but one (the subject) does not necessarily have to be aware of it. For negative capability to work its effects, the subject may not need Cartesian agency, so to speak. This is, in itself, no-knowledge, but yet a knowledge of which one cannot speak, which is the paradox of *Docta Ignorantia*, a necessarily incomplete project.

The next chapter will take a more in-depth look at the interviews and discuss them in relation to the general theme of the schema outlined here – *Docta Ignorantia*.

Endnotes

1. Some interviewees told me they liked X, Y, Z (e.g., house meetings, having house therapists, having time, etc.) and that these were helpful for their recovery, whilst *other* interviewees told me they disliked these things and they were unhelpful. There was no rhyme or reason or overarching theory that could be drawn out of such contradictions. Indeed, if quantitative statistical meta-analyses were carried out on 'communities and mental health' or even comparative qualitative meta-analyses, and such analyses ascertained 'trends' of significant therapeutic efficacy on the basis of the mode (most occurring so-called most liked and helpful factor of living in a community), the danger from a treatment planning approach would be that services could be moulded to fit such a finding. However, just because people 'dislike' some aspect of a community does not in itself mean that unhelpful qualities are unhelpful. The data in this study highlighted this paradox very well.

2. The reference to negative capability refers to the poet Keats, a practitioner of *Docta Ignorantia* who, in a letter to his brother in 1817, wrote: 'I had not a dispute but a disquisition with Dilke, on various subjects; several things dovetailed in my mind, and at once it struck me, what quality went to form a Man of Achievement especially in Literature and which Shakespeare possessed so enormously – I mean Negative Capability, that is when man is capable of being in uncertainties, Mysteries, doubts, without any irritable reaching after fact and reason …' (Gittings, *Selected Poems and Letters of Keats*, 1966, pp. 40–42).

Chapter Twenty

The honesty of the perplexed and the honesty of perplexity: Analysis of interviews

Ian Almond (2004) argues that confusion – from the etymological standpoint – means to make things flow together and to remove the borders, boundaries and distinctions which separate things into different categories. Confusion or bewilderment occurs when we come to the realisation that the rational intellect or ratiocination is not sufficient to comprehend what is occurring. Almond argues that confusion takes place because we insist on grasping onto something which veils us to what is actually going on. Neither Ibn 'Arabi (see Chittick, 1989) nor Jacques Derrida (see Derrida, 2007), in their respective philosophies, shy away from confusion or bewilderment; in fact it is a desirable and courageous state. Indeed, Heidegger took a similar stance. Heidegger explained that when something goes awry – an accident, one's partner leaves, projects fail – it is then we see how our world is structured and contextualised and how this gives one meaning. It is in this moment of 'breakdown' that we glimpse the worldhood of the world, as Heidegger coined it (Heidegger, 2001).

Hopefully the seeds of relevance of these ideas for the present project in relation to the interviewees' narratives are becoming apparent. In the philosophy of Heidegger (2001), and especially so in the Sufism of Ibn 'Arabi (Chittick, 1989) and the deconstructive thought of Derrida (2007), a common thread emerges: metaphysics (or medico-empirical-scientific ideas of mental distress) veils us from the actual situation. Therefore, if bewilderment or confusion (which is in opposition to the psycho-scientistic enterprise) disables our rationalising and desire for a system, structure or taxonomy, and we learn to desire this confusion, not to run away from it, then we will be able to 'see'. This is a paradox and a paradox not readily embraced by the medico-scientific community and their ideas of mental distress and how to deal with it. But I believe these ideas came through in the interviews with ex-residents.

Diana

Diana, our first interviewee, illustrates this paradox whilst also upholding Derrida's (2007) and Levinas's (2007) ethic of otherness or difference.

> Diana: *There is no us and them* [residents and house therapists] ... *of course there is an us and them ... you're there as a resident with issues, your therapist comes in and you know ... Acknowledge there is an us and them. That does not mean someone is superior or better. It acknowledges in fact there is a difference. Living in the houses can be extremely stressful at times and at times there is not enough support in the PA houses. I mean you're trying to work through your own shit and then you also have to deal with everyone else's shit.*

Diana then goes on to show how the ambience of having experts come into the houses (house therapists) does not degenerate into the therapist being able to 'tell residents how to get better' but instead upholds the equality and lets the 'otherness' of herself and her fellow residents be. She also alludes to one having to be confronted with one's 'own shit', to hit rock bottom, perhaps indicating the need not to shy away from the difficulty one faces.

> Diana: *... I think sometimes some people who go into the communities don't have the capacity. They have not hit rock bottom with the psychiatric services.*

> BS: Do you mean the people who go into the PA communities who have not hit rock bottom?

> Diana: *Yes ... some people have, some have not* [hit rock bottom]. *And I think generally ... if you have not hit rock bottom or if you haven't seen what the world has to offer in terms of support, you can't value what's different and you still might fight and kick against it but that's part of the process and I guess that's why I went in vowing I was going to make a difference ... that I didn't want to continue my life like this ... you know life was pretty shit and the world doesn't ... I mean even now it's bullshit ... people say there is more openness to people that have or has had mental*

> *health problems and that's crap ... and the PA houses do make an effort to normalise ...*
>
> *... They [people, prospective residents, the lay public] don't understand therapy, they don't understand that actually the houses are going to be hell, but you have to want to make a difference in your life and that's when it becomes difficult and the house is fractured in that sense. It's very hard. You always have people at different stages but you have to have people at the same starting point ... which is: I am going to make a difference to my life for real.*

It feels from Diana's comments that she became more aware of the difficulties that encroached upon her life and the inevitability of certain distasteful aspects that were actually real and very apparent. She seems to be of the idea that one has to be confronted with the bad aspects of society and also one has to be drawn down into despair to find one's way out.

The next excerpt from Diana's interview needs no explanation and speaks directly to the Derrida's (2007) and Ibn 'Arabi's (Chittick, 1989) ideals of bewilderment and confusion being a necessary evil.

> Diana: *You have to go through hell to find your way out ... it's your own personal hell, you can tell people it's actually going to happen but it's [telling them] not going to make a difference. However, they do need some preparation. I once had a therapist tell me this doesn't happen because most people would not go into it, because some people won't last if they knew the truth of the matter. Then they are not ready for therapy. If they are not ready for individual therapy, then they are not ready for the houses. It works, but it needs to be more realistic or it needs to be thought about more realistically about what it really is. That there are times when it does not work, and that is what sometimes makes it a success and completely unbearable to live in. I've been to hell and back and it was fantastic! The ultimate result is fantastic, but I would never choose to do that journey again. I hope that's been useful.*

Roland

Similar sentiments of bewilderment and confusion were expressed by Roland. More importantly, Roland's understanding of his experience, by being overly defined by his ex-therapist and the psychiatric hospital staff was, I feel, an effort by these professional helpers to banish confusion and a desire to gain clarity too quickly in a thoughtless way.

BS: ... what I am trying to say is, what was the thing that was therapeutic about being in the PA house, what is it that goes on in the house that is therapeutic and also is different from a hospital setting? What is it that you can identify as the process that goes on in the house?

Roland: *I mean, they are really difficult questions. Again I do sometimes wonder if I needed to be in the house ... I just felt safe when I arrived. I know I felt safe there because I felt as though ... because the fact that there were therapists coming in I thought well if people do treat me badly and if anything does happen to me then at least I have got a couple of therapists coming in. So I thought they are going to protect me or help me. So that was the kind of structure. Again I had people in the* [psychiatric] *hospital saying to me we think you have had too much psychotherapy and that actually it would be good for you not to have therapy now. So again there was this kind of ... when I was mentioning to people that I was thinking of moving into a therapeutic community, people were saying at the hospital, you have had enough therapy now. It's quite interesting because my therapist at the time said to me that I have told your story, you are ready to finish therapy now and I told him that I still feel absolutely crap.*

... I mean I remember one day my old therapist who was a clinical psychologist said to me 'I think you are depressed, let's get the DSM-III', and he was looking under the topic of depression and now when I think about it, I thought hang on a minute, he was performing to me ... it felt like a bit of a performance ... whether you use the DSM or not, it was the way he was flicking through the DSM ... 'Yes, you have got this, you have got this, and this.' he said. He said, 'I think you are depressed you know. I think you should go to your GP and get some antidepressants' ... I mean he is still around now. He still teaches now. I think he is quite a good therapist, but he screwed up with me though.

BS: So you left this guy, and did the therapists in the PA house kind of encourage you in a different direction to get another therapist?

Roland: *They put me in a different direction and the other thing is that I said that I felt crap and I've been told I had told my whole story and then (a house therapist) put me onto this analyst and the stuff that started flowing and I started coming out with this stuff. It was like having an orgasm and all this stuff started coming out, free association stuff and it felt absolutely wonderful to me.*

The idea of transcending symbolic boundaries in a positive sense – affirming subjectivity – comes through here, which is in line with Derrida's (1997) notion of deconstruction. Roland was allowed to break through boundaries, create, experiment, not be constrained, unlike his experience with the psychiatric system and his ex-therapist who defined Roland's situation. This lack of dogmatism by the PA setup was elaborated upon by him later in our conversation.

Roland: *They* [the house therapists] *certainly did not coerce me in any way. I remember having this sense from (the house therapists) whatever I said, people agreed with. This felt quite new to me because I spent a large part of my life saying things and people disagreeing with me. So I have always assumed that I am wrong ... So that was the thing about the house; people did agree with me and this was new for me. But then the other thing was that I saw the PA house as just a normal house. Even though the therapists came in we certainly did not have formal group psychotherapy. I mean it did feel more like living in a family. The love that I felt from (the house therapists) ... .and when I say love it's kind of just the acceptance ... it was far more powerful on a deeper level than I had experienced before.*

The above passage from Roland's interview conjures up the idea of Roland being let free to meander in his narrative, being received by the other residents. I feel they certainly would not have agreed with *all* of what Roland said, but at the very least, it seems, they let him have his say, be heard and witnessed. This was also, it seems, encouraged by the house therapists by not imposing Lacan's (2007) discourse of the master (i.e., not imposing a kind of formal group therapy treatment with the therapists as masters and controllers).

Roland's references to a family and love are very interesting. For a human being to flourish, to have 'room' to move about freely and be given acceptance of their meanderings and creativities, is what one expects in a good-enough loving family setup. Of course one may make mistakes, but part of growing (and growing up, especially in ordinary families) necessitates making mistakes, forgiveness, repentance, and carrying on in such ordinariness and uncertainty. This structure seems present in Roland's narrative; there is not a lot of certainty regarding his outcome and struggle with his mental distress, but there is a space to move. Of course, such a structure (or structure-less-ness) was not apparent with his experience of his previous therapist (see above) and his stay in a psychiatric hospital.

> Roland: ... But ... everybody stays away from you when you go into hospital. All the staff go into this office. It's like a glass house. You see all the staff in this glass room, all staying with themselves. They all look terrified to come out of this glass room. And there is you as a patient and there is all these mad people running up and down the ward completely naked and you're thinking, I ought to be in that glass room where they are safe ... it's very strange ... very strange. To see people in that situation ... but I mean more or less, they just leave you to yourself. Nobody talks to you; nobody wants to really listen to you. So you are just left to your own devices. They give you something to help you sleep at night ... its bizarre, bizarre... Most of the psychiatrists see the patient maybe once all the time they are in there. It's quite bizarre how people want to go in.

Returning to the theme of the ordinariness and the inevitable mystery of everyday life as both Derrida and Ibn 'Arabi would attest to (see Almond, 2004), one has to learn to accept some kind of mystery and bewilderment in life to live it. To cordon off life into neat little packages would be detrimental to a feeling of being alive. Even after leaving the house, Roland still feels (at times) bewildered, but is able to stay with this. This marks an important difference between people who get hopelessly lost trying to cure their 'mental illness' and those who can (non-)manage with their distress in a non-grasping, panic-free way. This was expressed by Roland towards the end of the interview.

Roland: *I don't see myself as a success story as somebody who has left the house. I don't feel that I am a good person to talk to about the houses. OK I have left and I am still struggling, but I guess who is not struggling. So I see somebody like (X)*[an ex-resident of a PA house]; *she is a success. But that might be my biased perception. I have always shared mostly* [lived in shared houses] *and have only lived on my own twice and here for about three years. So I can live on my own but I don't see that as a success story. Often I think I have done all this therapy just to live on my own. It does not seem to make sense. I missed the house when I first moved out and I missed the sense of belonging to a group of people. Coming home there, there was always a sense of something happening. So again when I lived in the house I thought I can't wait till I get my own place and now that I have got my own place I think it would be lovely to be with other people.*

Joe

I propose that a closing down of exploring beyond predetermined boundaries is what makes up much of the 'state's' and medico-scientific community's ideology about mental distress – prescribed ways of doing things (i.e., NICE guidelines, Health and Care Professions Council, Improving Access to Psychological Therapies (IAPT), CBT etc.), which are thoughtlessly adopted by many people. Demarcation is carried out; the territory (e.g., human cognition or mental illness) is claimed in an imperial and totalitarian fashion and CBT or drugs are heralded as the new 'Promised Land'. But inevitably, this restricts movement and blocks 'the flow' on many levels. Joe, a veteran of three PA communities, explained in a beautiful and succinct way how such flows are stopped or diverted.

Joe: *... The whole cause is something I still do believe in. I don't think about it all that much, but it is nice to know ... 40 years on and it's still causing controversy and people are still questioning what it means to be mad and what it means to be sane and what it means to be free.*

... I was an enfant terrible and at the end of the day infants have to grow up and I don't know whether my time in the houses was part of being childish and that the responsible adult thing to do was to have nothing to do with that ... I don't know ... it's taught me things I can't

put into words ... I would do it again, I would do it again but, I am not sure whether there is much of an opportunity to do anything like that again. As you say it's very much the question of just two houses now ... I think for me it was part of growing up for a very immature boy, into a more solidly based thinking person ... it was a second childhood because my first one was such a mess ... I needed a second one. I watched a TV programme about the Clouds rehab centre and a girl was talking about having been given a great opportunity and I thought ... very few people are given the opportunity to express themselves exactly as they want ... and I thought, hang on a minute ... I had that opportunity and it is a very rare precious thing that I have been given and she is right .. we live in a very regimented society and she said the ability to be just yourself which she experienced at the rehab centre. She pointed out very few people are granted that and I thought I was given that, I was granted that. I must count myself very, very fortunate to have been given such a wonderful opportunity and be careful not to waste it, which is why I am very pleased to have talked to you today. You know I want my experience to count for something, because very few people are given the opportunity I had and it just doesn't happen in most people's lives.

Rob

As I mentioned at the beginning of this chapter, when outlining Derrida's and Ibn 'Arabi's (Almond, 2004; Derrida, 1997; Chittick, 1989) ideas in relation to the present project, I talked about the danger of imperialistic system building and the futility of cordoning off 'aspects' of human experience. Tying in these ideas with the ideas of Parmenides reveals an interesting unveiling; the problematic of veiling aspects of human experience and making these aspects, things that *are*, not seem to be. However, as Parmenides explained more than 2,500 years ago, such ideas, of making things, human experience or ideas into *non-being*, are just not possible (see Kingsley, 1999; Geldard, 2007; Heidegger, 1998). In our contemporary psychiatric/psychological system-building world, many things are cast out[1] as they are regarded as not belonging within the territory enclosed within their taxonomies (or ignored as they are regarded as not being valid as a territory). It is fair to say, to deduce from this, that a risk of banishing 'aspects' and stopping or diverting flows may lead to inauthenticity, or turning away from truthfulness or at the very least ignoring certain aspects of it (Deleuze & Guattari, 2004). I felt from Rob's descriptions (see below) that the PA houses encourage everything to come into the mix, as it were, where a vibrancy or aliveness is the result.

> Rob: ... *And I liked the whole spirit of the house. People would sit there and have a go at you. There was something very real about it, something very raw. It felt like there was something really going on there and I really quite enjoyed that. The energy was very high; not like the previous place* [a therapeutic community] *I lived. There was not the same energy or focus on therapy there as there was in the PA ...*
>
> *... Living in the house was a fucking nightmare. It was also very powerful and helpful. I wish I could sit here and give you a tidy response. In some way I miss the rawness of it and the real struggle to be honest* [the effort of being honest]. *When I had your email I kind of got excited because I had not had any contact with the PA for about two years. It is, the experience of the houses, is something that I have not experienced outside the houses. It was tremendously rich and it was a mixture of total fucking boredom, growth, and transformation all mixed up together ...*
>
> *That really got me moving and woke me up ... in a way that I had not realised to the other residents ...*
>
> *... The therapists were all kind of from the late 60s and they like broke every fucking rule in the book and I think they were quite brilliant, quite brilliant and it was what I liked about the houses ... is that they* [the house therapists] *would take risks and they would go off ... they wouldn't just cover their own backs, they would take risks and break the rules ...*
>
> *... I feel so incredibly grateful. I feel I was able to function and move on and you know, not be a mental case despite the fact I still have ongoing problems but I am still in therapy but they sort of went to an effort. They* [the PA house therapists] *didn't worry too much about following some stupid guidebook to cover their own backs. You really felt they were doing what they could to help you. It was a very strange experience and I will always be grateful.* [Rob at this point was very tearful, in a joyful way.]

Julia

The more authentic environment that can exist in a PA house was also echoed by Julia, and reasons why such environments are being cordoned off, out of existence.

> Julia: *From what I have seen of mental health services as an adult personally, and professionally* [in her job within the mental health field] *there was a family and community atmosphere that wasn't clinical; a more natural way to help people heal. People were encouraged to get on and do things for themselves, make stuff, fix things, grow their own food. I've seen this in a watered-down version on psychiatric wards with OT* [occupational therapy] *sessions, they are more like add-ons; patients don't cook their own dinner, they have cooking lessons or sessions. They don't build stuff for the ward or their home; they make a piece of arts and crafts that is expressive, but separate from real life. There needs to be a crossover, some kind of middle ground I think, to keep people attached to reality.*
>
> *... I think that the PA house I stayed in was of its time ... nowadays people are more afraid, authorities are scared of being sued if things go wrong and are only interested in providing the bare minimum at the least cost. There seems to be no quality of care. 'Community care' just doesn't seem to work, there are a lot of isolated people out there suffering from mental health difficulties.*

Julia's interview touches upon a very thoughtful issue highlighting how so-called caring-community contexts (i.e., psychiatric care in an outreach context) and the care psychologists and psychotherapists strive for in trying to help, cure, alleviate, and one must say, normalise everyone to be the same (i.e., happy, mentally healthy, sane, etc.), miss a very important facet of human life: the extraordinary, the mysterious, the unknown, or the *uncanny* as Heidegger (2001) would say.

Heidegger (1998), drawing on the philosophy of Parmenides,[2] describes that when being comes into focus, the extraordinary announces itself, the excessive that strays beyond the ordinary, that which cannot be explained by explanations of the basis of beings. In other words, Heidegger argues that the uncanny cannot be measured at all within the measure of the standard. The uncanny is the simple, the insignificant, and ungraspable by the will and by the artifices of calculative thought. The uncanny is everywhere at all times. Heidegger's ideas obviously mirror

Ibn 'Arabi's and Derrida's doubts about system building (see Almond, 2004) and Lacan's (2006) notion of the ungraspable Real.

Simon

These ideas are pertinent to the interview of Simon. I feel in many ways that Simon exemplified, and I do not mean in any way for this to sound derogatory, our present culture's need to explain and normalise mental distress, and also to find a cure so to speak. One example of this would be the utopian revolution of cognitive behavioural therapy and the historical emergence of the government's Improving Access to Psychological Therapies programme (IAPT). This has helped to instil in many people the idea that their mental distress can be normalised solely within these systems, and if they fail (i.e., to get the person cured), there must be something else to be done and/or there must be something wrong with the person seeking relief. This is a very precarious discourse to entertain. As Simon stated:

> Simon: ... *I could not understand why* [I was distressed] *and so I went into the PA house to help with this and my social communication problems to find out about my psychological blocks and if anything could be done to remove them. But that never happened in the ten months I was there.*

Simon clearly entertains the ideas of 'blocks' in his psyche, and that there should be, within the context of the PA house 'treatment', something occurring or being done to him, and within a certain amount of time (ten months), these blocks should have been taken away. As Heaton (2010) eloquently points out, such a way of thinking about the mind leads us down rabbit holes and to conceptual riddles that lead us far from a path of truthfulness: i.e., mystifying ideas about mental functioning and meta-psychology. This conceptually faulty thinking is revered in the mental health world and is drip-fed via various media into people's consciousness. Another consequence is that 'theorists' in the field breed 'masters' of knowledge on wellbeing that we become enslaved to. This is of such insidiousness that it creeps into one's narrative, resulting in the asking of impossible questions. As Simon describes:

> Simon: *Well when I once saw a trainee psychotherapist she seemed to know a lot about me before I even told her much about me from what I explained about what my parents were like. And I never found that from*

> *the therapists in the house. Or maybe because I never spoke much in the house meetings. That's the only difference that I can think of. They never had as much insight into me as I would have liked ...*
>
> *... I just wished that I had spoken a lot more. I just wish that the house therapists had had more insight into me and said things like my old psychotherapist like ... unconscious stuff to do with my family. My old psychotherapist told me that my parents' strange behaviour was due to their childhood. I am convinced if they* [the house therapists] *had had more insight into me they would have been able to help me.*
>
> *... Maybe a combination of psychotherapy and CBT* [is needed in the PA houses] *so people can change their negative and irrational beliefs. Because otherwise you have got to work it out for yourself. Like my old therapist said to me, 'How can I conquer this?', I mean even if you accept it, so I did. How can I work it out, how can I think differently?*

To be fair to Simon, perhaps he didn't spend enough time in the house and/or it was just not for him – and that is reasonable. But he did get some benefit from the house and did feel that the house offered something valuable. Simon told me a few months after the interview had taken place that he felt that if he had given the house more time (i.e., stayed longer) that the therapists and living in the house could have helped him even more.

> Simon: *I started to like the people there immediately, but as I said, the house never solved this problem I had with communication. But being there did help me with my paranoia about not being liked or being disrespected ... I realised that I was liked and respected by the other residents to some degree.*

> BS: So do you think it helped you with some aspects of your self-esteem?

> Simon: *Self-esteem ... yes. Yes ... you see I was not sleeping properly, concentrating properly, I was confused. I had a problem with my blood, I thought it was. I was worrying too much and drinking in the evenings. Then I found out what was wrong and the doctor gave me medication for*

high blood pressure or something. So I am not totally better now but I am a lot better now. I left under a cloud of confusion; I threatened another resident and said I would hit him. I left that same night, but I later apologised to him.

... My self-esteem went up, the house helped that.

BS: Do you think there was any particular reason why the house did this? What do you think it was?

Simon: *Living with other people. Not being frightened of having problems, not being frightened of [being] judged as being psychological. So living with other people helped me. I tried my best to support and understand them, they did their best to support and understand me.*

... I just wished that I had spoken a lot more.

Sally

The interview with Simon made me think that he was attempting to contain his distress within a boundary, and was trying to stop himself from breaking through this boundary by 'not getting into the house'. This is interesting considering the next interview with Sally, where all boundaries of her distress were, it seems, in the context of the PA house, torn asunder, and causing a reconfiguration of the past, where previously she and her mental health professionals had attempted to contain the distress within a rigid discourse or framework; this unsurprisingly had failed, leaving her in a place of bewilderment and perplexity.

Sally: *Just before I was looking at (PA house) I was in a crisis. I had reached a point where I wanted to do something quite ... I needed to make a big change ... I knew I wanted to live with other people ... but knew it needed to be a supportive environment ... I had been living on my own and so I was very isolated and I was living with a woman who took me in out of kindness of her heart really. I had been working part time for over a year ... but then I just completely broke down, and I stopped working. I was just in a bit of a mess really. I was just looking for a fresh start. But that was ... I had had a long, long history of mental health issues since I was a child.*

Soon after moving into the house, Sally was faced with having to deal with this bewilderment and negotiate its territory, and tackle the frustration of not being helped in a way which would shore up this bewilderment, in a way which she imagined would rectify this. However, it could be argued that all her previous experiences in the mental health world were undoubtedly fuelled by the discourse of enclosing, classifying, and attempting to solve her problems. Her PA house experience seemed not to repeat the previous failures, or the false or misguided hope common to psychiatric discourse.

> Sally: *I found it very hard to use them* [the house meetings] *to begin with. I was terrified and I would often just sit and I didn't feel able to participate and I would often go in with my little piece of paper with things written down that I wanted to say but I didn't manage to say. I was kind of wanting people to help me to sort of ... you know ... get into the meetings. But that was rarely the case and certainly the therapists didn't make any effort.*

Indeed, Sally's reliance and placing of importance upon the psychiatric discourse was highlighted later on during the interview and how she found it very disconcerting that the house therapists didn't place much importance on the psychiatric label, as though such an enclosure/label was necessary for her, or should be.

> Sally: ... *he* [her psychiatrist] *dealt with my medication ... I discovered after a few months of moving to London that I had been diagnosed with (a psychiatric disorder) ... I was never told this before. Apparently this was written in my notes by my psychiatrist without anybody telling me anything. I was very shocked they would do that. I remember I went back to a meeting* [the PA house meeting] *and told them that my psychiatrist told me that I have (a psychiatric disorder),* [and that] *it was written in my notes and ... the house therapists were very nonplussed about it really ... and I was like ... do I have this? ... do I have it? ... and somehow it was important that I had been given this label.*

The irony of her situation, in wanting people to tell her how to be, how to get well, and explain her experience for her, which might have inadvertently reinforced her previously failed attempts at healing, is that she found her own way; she came to her own 'mind' about what should occur. She became confident in what path to take, and less dependent on what others thought.

> Sally: *It was really learning to live with other people ... it was really, really good ... it was hard but ... just for me, learning about social interaction ... it was quite important and in the end I kind of felt like to me it was good for me to stop and see that actually these meetings didn't help me or at least they don't help me anymore and I actually don't agree with this you know ... the way that the therapists were working and for me to actually stand up and say this isn't what I want ... I want to move on was really important for me ... to make that decision ... but I have very mixed feelings about the whole experience really but I don't totally regret it. Coming to London gave me that fresh start I needed and for me getting the space from where I grew up and my family and everything was really good. And trying to learn how to speak during the meetings, what I felt about things. But what I think really benefited me more was from what other residents in the house said, more than what the therapists said.*

The idea of making up her own 'mind' was reiterated later on during the interview.

> BS: Interesting ... so you became frustrated with this state of affairs [in the house] and you felt you had to make your own mind up and just go for it despite what others thought?

> Sally: *Yeah ... yeah ... but in some ways for me that was quite good ... it gave me more confidence ... to think actually this is what I want to do ... and you know I am actually going to do it ... despite the fact that you* [the house therapists] *don't agree ... I was terrified to say that* [to the house therapists] *but I did ... and you know I do feel that I absolutely made the right decision to go there* [the PA house] *at the time and make the* [correct] *decision to leave when I did.*

> BS: Sounds like it's a bit of a paradox really?

> Sally: *It is really ... because I don't want to totally say I don't like the*

house, [that] it didn't do me any good or anything, because it was not like that. I don't want to come over as if it was all negative, but for me there were a lot of negative things but not everything.

Sally's interview again highlights some very important points; chaos (or lack of structure) and lack of clarity of the road ahead, leading to a paradox. Of course there is something implicitly negative about this notion – a breakdown in structure – but this can be positive, as a breakdown of structure unveiling the paradoxes, or deconstruction to use Derrida's terminology, can be fruitful (see Derrida, 1982, 1997, 2004). Derrida describes how deconstruction, with its effects of *Différance*[3] and dissemination, is bewildering (Derrida, 1982, 1997, 2004). *Différance* is anarchic, it instigates the subversion of every kingdom, and it escapes and disorganises structure, deconstructs the text unsews it, and explodes the semantic horizon of the subject. To relate these ideas to our present purpose, *Différance*, whilst it confuses things, can make things simple; it breaks downs complexities, totalisations, or over-simplifications (e.g., the theory of negative cognitions associated with CBT, getting happiness, being cured from mental illness, or how to live in a community; deconstruction calls these *concepts*, *ideas*, and *strategies* into question). It dismantles structures (i.e., lived, and oppressive structures); for example, the capitalist demand that one must be a successful producer, be happy, successful, sociable, and sane. In other words, although it may make things difficult to understand, if there are no actual real dichotomies of negative and positive cognitions, sane/insane way to live etc., then *Différance* takes away the intended or primary sense of a structure (e.g., deconstructing the idea that CBT creates happy cognitions or the therapeutic techniques of how to live, or be cured when living in a community). However, in taking away the primary sense (or at least holding it into question, as oppressive) this opens up the 'text' for other senses, other directions.

Although some may shudder, without the rudder (of structure) to guide and place upon a way, it is not Derrida's (1997, 2004) intention via his argument of deconstruction to make things more confusing; on the contrary, Derrida wants to show how the text (or structure) is in itself actually confused. Thus deconstruction is an act of revelation. The drifting of the text or structure precedes any theoretical intervention; within a text or structure, there is always drifting. Although deconstruction might be assumed to create chaos, in actual fact a deconstructive process shows how these uncontrollable elements (within so-called calm, serene, untroubled texts or structures) are actually full of contradiction and instability. Confusion, perplexity, and instability are part of every text; it does not matter if such a text has been subjected to analysis or not. Thus confusion and perplexity, especially in relation to the text or structure of something called a cure, treatment, taxonomy or theory for mental illness, are inevitable. Such confusion or perplexity may or may not fuel and drive the desire to the truer, more confused state of things and not to surrender to looking for a secure system. These are important points in relation to the next interview with Thomas which I will now discuss.

Thomas

The PA in the early history of the community was very much fuelled by the ethos coined by Laing: 'Everything is up for grabs' (see Mullan, 1995). Of course this was a subversive and deconstructive gesture, and one of the PA communities' most famous residents, Mary Barnes (see Mullan, 1995), was an example of deconstruction, regressing to the state of a baby, to go down, to die and to be reborn and come out the other side. Her story appealed to the dissatisfaction of those in society who opposed and questioned the oppressive nature of psychiatric discourse and treatment of the day. Thomas commented on this appeal and deconstructive praxis of living in a PA community.

> Thomas: *I felt the PA houses were probably more open and congenial to some people's way of living, after having been influenced by the story of Mary Barnes and the fact that I had seen the film about the Archway Community where Leon Redler was and other people ...* Asylum, *that was the film ... so that was my motivation to go into the houses ...*
>
> *... I had to adjust in a house which turned day into night and night into day. So breakfast was around lunch or maybe after lunch ... maybe 2pm or 3pm. It was then people got up and started moving around the house; some silent, some chatty, and then life started to warm up around 5pm or 6pm where lunch would get cooked. Dinner was sometime around 10.30pm to 11pm. So my whole structure of time and rhythm was turned not quite upside-down but turned around – that's the concept of autorhythmia, we could follow our own rhythm ...*
>
> *... in the evening there was some warmth and discussion and sometimes arguments; lots of smoking ... lots of smoking and endlessly drinking and debates and imagination ... and Ronnie* [Laing] *this and Ronnie that* [people talking about Laing] *... Some people were more open or closed or congenial than others.*

> ... It was freer to be in a PA house than say in the (another previous non-PA community), which I experienced before and [in the PA house] there was no staff/patient distinction directly on a day-to-day level. But it was of course clear to all in the house that people staying there who were training therapists were training therapists and people who were patients were wholly patients ... But it was also a bit mystifying.

But in this chaos that Thomas describes there seemed to be, as Derrida describes is essential in a deconstructive process, a need for courage and honesty in trying to find one's own way, rather than being told to submit to a structure, which may have been constricting and knotting up of any sense of being able to go beyond the text. Thomas describes this struggle in a positive way on one hand, as unhelpful on the other, but seemingly paradoxically helpful as well; leading him to seek help with one of the house therapists. Even Laing himself, as shown from Thomas's description (see below) demonstrated this *way* to a good and positive effect. Such demonstrations in today's culture by 'mental health professionals' would be frowned upon. Indeed, from the standards set by the Health and Care Professions Council for psychologists, any mental health issues or problems identified in a practitioner psychologist could be used as evidence as being 'unfit to practise'.[4]

> Thomas: *Another thing in comparison to other places; there was the autorhythmia. We did not have rigid structures except the community meeting. The rest was up for grabs. One could of course if one went to meeting, one would not turn up late.*
>
> *... But in the house there was nothing set and of course in the (non-PA therapeutic community where Thomas had lived for a period of time previously) everybody cooked, shopped, and participated. In the PA there were also drawing classes and yoga. So there were some structure and time, but generally it was very free. For some people it was more helpful to have a clear structure and for some people it was clear to have very little structure, and very little support. I mean some people were really begging for support and asking for support which they then got from members of the PA. Of course one had to own up to one's own voice.*
>
> *... I also found helpful that I was challenged in the house in regards my own inner assumptions about how to live a good life and how to live*

together and see and be in doubt and to enlarge my tolerance, my ability to be tolerant.

So that's what I found helpful. Also the humour and the fun we had together in the house like when Ronnie [Laing] *came round for a meeting, after the house meeting was over he made a contribution of whisky and he would join in and drink and smoke hashish. So that was part of the ritual when the big master would come round. We would have great fun and a celebration. He* [Laing] *would talk a bit and sometimes he would show up especially after his daughter Susie died and he would show us how sad he was, and how we could use the households to express ourselves ... when we are in dire straits in moments in our lives. Showing; that's what Ronnie* [Laing] *did and I appreciated his teaching by example.*

... [what he found unhelpful in the house was] *the lack of a daily structure, the lack of a daily ritual, the lack of real presence of therapists in the house, of giving a certain hold and warmth in the house.*

... [how he remedied this and what he found helpful] *what I found helpful was the clarity which I got from (a PA house therapist) who was for me the only one besides Ronnie, who I could always approach and make an appointment with if I wanted to. (The PA house therapist) said my door is always open; you can come by if you need some help, please approach me and speak things out. So I found this very good. He became my elder brother in a sense but also sometimes I found him to be more like a father figure.*

Interestingly, as Derrida (1997) would describe, a deconstructive approach takes courage and therefore it may not be for everyone. From Thomas's descriptions, this rings true for the PA community house experience. However, it seemed there were different houses offering different things for different people; people with different needs, desires, aims, goals and abilities. But importantly, this did not seem to be a prearranged plan on the part of the PA. Therapists of different orientations are/were 'allowed' to practise in their own way and also find their own autorhythmia which unsurprisingly was one reason which helped potential residents choose which house they wished to apply to live in based on how it felt to them; how the therapists seemed to be to them.

Thomas: *Not for everyone* [the PA houses] *I must say. If one could have the PA the way it is now, or the way it was in the past one could say maybe go to different houses which catered for different kinds of people, to see what they are like. We had this; houses catering for different types of people and distress and we also had different types of therapists in the different houses.*

David

David echoed Thomas's and other interviewees' sentiment that living in a PA house was a difficult and challenging place to be. Too often reports of a 'treatment' being difficult and challenging within the sphere of 'mental health' is often deemed faulty, ineffective, dangerous, not meeting an individual's or organisation's 'duty of care', and this is often one reason that drives instances of complaint and litigation. Such a view is obviously a one-sided view and omits, banishes, covers up, and forgets the possibility of a Derridean deconstructive movement (Derrida, 1997). Often a deconstructive movement is extremely difficult or intangible to grasp, formulate, or speak about in a contemporary academic, theoretical, and logical way. Indeed a deconstructive movement is what I feel I have witnessed from listening to my interviewees, and this deconstructive practice seems to be the praxis of the houses – a praxis that generates a movement or nomadic current that moves beyond systems or system building, states, taxonomies and outcomes. But to initiate or get involved in this praxis, as Derrida (1997) describes, takes courage and great strength, and is by no means possible to do easily or without any pain and suffering. Such praxis also allows one to call into question the role of the expert or the professional of mental distress; something that in our contemporary situation is hardly entertained. David describes this painful and thoughtful praxis eloquently and how it was helpful.

David: *The house was though a very difficult place to live. I found it very hard living there …*

… So it was very hard. I was doing my very best to follow that regime but I found it incredibly difficult, stressful and quite exhausting. The meetings themselves were often quite fraught. There was a lot of going on about I suppose quite trivial things, quite little things between people that would get talked about and more often than not I felt they were getting escalated rather than any sort of light being shed upon what was going on.

At the same time there was a feeling of emotional connection between us, so there was a sense of us being part of something even though we were at each other's throats. I think there was a sense of intimacy there. We did all talk about very difficult and painful things from our pasts as well in quite an open manner which I think did lead us into a connection between us.

... I was challenged. I think it gave me an opportunity to see very young childish parts of myself which I think I was quite ashamed of and not very much in touch with and quite resistant to exploring. But they obviously played themselves out [with] *other people in the house. That was something that was brought up in the meetings. So although I found that difficult and painful, I think it was quite helpful. I talked a lot about relationships. That was my difficulty with personal relationships, especially sexual relationships with the opposite sex. That was something that was a big difficulty for me. It was good to talk with other people who experienced the same difficulties as well. I think I found that enormously helpful; to talk about relationships and sex and those sorts of things. I found that very, very helpful;* [having] *very deep, intimate, and quite profound conversations with people in and out of the meetings, which I found enormously uplifting. I mean first of all, just the process of just acknowledging just how crap inside I really did feel, which took a while because I was quite well defended I think, but in a fairly kind of sophisticated way. Then having acknowledged that it was very useful for me to realise that pretty much, we are all in the same boat. The symptoms and the ways it affected our lives ... I think we* [David and the other residents] *were very different as individuals, our personalities were all very different. But I think there was an underlying understanding. Something we* [David and the other residents] *have all shared in common as well which I found very helpful. I found the presence of the therapists very helpful as well. They were both very experienced and very compassionate people. I think they were certainly saner than my parents were. They didn't do my head in the same way that my parents did. They certainly did do my head in at times. I was never uncritical in my discussions with them but yeah, they helped enormously. They were role models to us to a certain extent, certainly to begin with.*

David had experienced psychiatric care, which as I have mentioned previously, focuses upon mental distress in a very non-Derridean way. Indeed, the challenging and the allowing of the challenging and questioning of one another and even the professional roles are banished in a psychiatric environment where the psychiatrist or doctor is master, and the patient is slave. Even though David was very critical of the PA house he lived in, he had these comments to share regarding his views on a PA house compared to a psychiatric hospital.

David: *Vastly superior* [the PA houses in comparison to psychiatric hospitals]. *I have been quite critical I think partly because if the houses are to survive and to flourish I would genuinely like to see them do that. I think it is important to see how they can do things better. But I suppose partly I am coming from the perspective of what the ideal house could be. However, when you compare the houses to, and I have had a fair amount of experience of this as well, the medical model, medication-based approach to mental illness, there is no doubt the houses are far superior ... I mean to me the houses prove that the medical model ... you know I have never believed the medical model of mental health. I never believed it was analogous to having high blood pressure or something like that; so you take pills the rest of your life for bipolar disorder or schizophrenia or whatever. I have never bought into that analogy. But I also think the house proved* [its effectiveness], *because I was a wreck when I went in there. I can't really express just what terrible shape physically* [I was in]; *the reality was that it was entirely due to psychological factors. It was entirely by addressing the psychological factors in the house and in my own therapy and yes in life outside, as I have carried on doing that my physical condition improved ... I think the house therapists were extremely helpful in linking explicitly to my psychology and not letting me off the hook on that issue. As a result I improved enormously and there is no doubt the basic process worked and you know I would be ... I don't really see how I could have managed without something like that. And I think hospital is appalling ... I couldn't live with my parents ... I could not be in hospital. Yes it was very different living in the house and I have a number of suggestions (laughs) in which it could be made easier, but it was still a hell of a lot better than any of the alternatives available that I know of. And I am quite passionate about the potential of what the houses can, could and should do. I think they are enormously helpful things. I do want to support them even though I had my difficulties there as I have said.*

Lastly, David again hinted towards the challenge involved in the Derridean movement and praxis involved.

David: *I feel as though I have utterly transcended the situation that I was in when I went into the house. That is also partly due to my own efforts since I came out the house, but that made it possible for me to get onto that foothold. So the house has taken me out of the NHS care altogether.*

Peter

I feel that Peter highlights the fact that Laing and the early PA personnel who set up Kingsley Hall and the early PA communities were aware of the gravity and wrong-footedness of running a PA community in line with a medicalised model. They realised how this would detract from a praxis of deconstruction that left open 'space' and created space (and time) for people living there to move freely, but also to be allowed to experience the gamut of their own and each other's experience without some form of closing down; i.e., from the oppression of the master–slave dialectic (psychiatrist–patient) and the thoughtless medico-scientific attempts to stop one's suffering, which inadvertently prevents one the valuable possibility of deconstructing past imaginary constructions and relationships with others, by staying with one's suffering. Peter's interview was also illuminating in debunking the myth that Laing and the Philadelphia Association would stop people having conventional psychiatric treatment and were 'anti-psychiatry'. Of course a Derridean deconstructive move would question such bracketing off of options or banishing ways, means, and options a person chooses in how he or she wanted to be treated; excluding choice does not seem to have been part of the ethos of the early PA communities nor the present-day PA houses.

Peter: *He didn't want people there because they were therapists. He wanted people who loved the ideas. He [Laing] said it was probably better if there were no doctors or psychologists here at all. He said he would have preferred if there were carpenters and washer women; these kinds of people had knowledge of human life and a love of people. That would be great he [Laing] said. But unfortunately a lot of people who were into psychology wanted to be there because they thought they would learn something, or maybe become famous . .*

... So that was my experience. Day-to-day life was what it was all about. So the therapy, I mean as someone often said, 'therapy is not something that should be consigned to the consulting room'. Therapy is going on all the time in one form or another, in one's life. So one shouldn't think it is a professional activity necessarily. It is the way the soul is met with by other people. Some ways are very destructive and devastating, other ways are the opposite ...

... 'We all need to learn to be a bit more mad.' He [Laing] *encouraged people who were there* [in the PA house] *who were not suffering or diagnosed with something, to just let go, to let their own madness come out. He did not say 'do and say mad crazy things', but 'just try to let go a bit' ...*

... Quite a few people who came to (the PA community house) who had come from a mental hospital and their psychiatrists had been giving them Largactil, Stelazine or something similar like that. They were meant to be taking the stuff; usually they would not bother after a while, but some of them had to report after a while [to their psychiatrist] *so they had to keep taking their drugs. There was not as much enforcement as there is today. It was a bit more lax. If you were not dangerous, you were left* [alone] *so Ronnie* [Laing] *never prescribed medication at all. I think sometimes he* [Laing] *would give someone a tranquilliser if the person was in a lot of distress but it was not the policy of the place. It was not an either/or, he was just saying why do we have to make people take drugs when they can get along with human contact? There was a lot of love in (the PA community house). A lot of caring and I think that Ronnie showed people that he cared by the way that he treated people, how he dealt with them ...*

... There was no policy as such like 'you should be on medication or you should not be' in those days. There was no kind of issue ...

Interestingly though, Peter described how with certain psychiatric drugs, the experience of taking them (i.e., anti-psychotic medication, Largactil) seemed conducive to preventing a deconstructive movement or praxis taking place.

> Peter: *... So I took it* [Largactil] *and I felt awful. It cuts you off like you're in cotton wool, you don't feel anything, you can't speak, you can't think, you're just in a daze; hopeless stuff. That was my one experience of Largactil.*

As mentioned previously the idea of 'going down', letting somebody go down into their madness, and the questioning of madness were somethings that Laing encouraged. This idea has obvious resonances with a Derridean deconstructive (Derrida, 1997) or nomadic movement (see Deleuze & Guattari, 2004), of not being constrained by a space or dwelling, ring-fenced off so to speak, or prevented from moving, but allowing a natural movement to take place and being able and supported to move into domains, which albeit painful and frightening, may let someone glimpse a truer state of affairs.

> Peter: *This* [going down] *was the one thing that was probably of uppermost importance for (the ethos of the PA community experience). Ronnie understood this very well, the importance of this. He* [Laing] *had experienced this as a young psychiatrist of having two or three patients described in* [Laing's] *the book* Wisdom, Madness and Folly. *They were young men who were in a mental hospital ... so he* [Laing] *invited them to come to his house and stay with his family. It was very daring and very courageous thing to do. So he had experience of somebody going to their room, going down and being quiet. For him, when he* [Laing] *visited the padded cells in the mental hospital, he would try to get them to calm down and talk, and usually they would be fine with him sitting in the padded cell; which was something nobody had done before.*

The idea of a deconstructive move present in the ethos of Peter's PA community house was further elaborated upon in the questioning of the role of the 'professional' helper. In other words the role of the imaginary, in the Lacanian sense (Lacan, 2006) of an ideal sane, trouble-free, and superior individual, was questioned, and how these ideas affected individuals and/or the praxis of the community as a whole. Of course, such a path is painful and challenging, but this constant flow of openings and closings was needed to prevent stagnation and totalising systems to occur.

> Peter: *I would say that alchemically I experienced the nigredo. I was going*

> *through a lot of difficult stuff, so to go somewhere for this to happen, to feel that I was part of something, the value of this type of experience was recognised. So some people who came there to work might have become quite superior, which the guy I mentioned earlier* [a therapist who worked at Peter's PA community house], *he became quite superior minded I think. Whereas, some people* [residents and people involved with the community] *became quite cynical with what they saw, people misusing, abusing the place, but to develop a nuance you have to see what is the misuse and what they are actually doing. You've got to point it out to them and get them to see their shadow or their aspect of their Nafs* [a Sufi term for egotistical behaviour]. *They have to see what they are doing which is causing distress or destruction, something about them that can't be criticised, about what they can't take criticism for, get them to see that they see that their way is the right way, but they are blind to the fact that they are being cruel, destructive, and mean.*

Towards the end of his interview Peter talked about contemporary society, with its reliance on a narrow scientific and technological ideology which he believed leaves little place for such endeavours that occurred in the early PA communities and in today's PA communities. Peter described how we are limited by the sense of linear progression in all spheres of life which imbues one with a false sense of foundation, banishing myth and mystery, or the real. As mentioned earlier, Parmenides believed banishing aspects to so-called non-existence was a very dangerous path to take; such aspects would not in fact disappear, but only continue to rumble and possibly erupt from the real (see Kingsley, 1999; Geldard, 2007; Heidegger, 1998).

> Peter: *There certainly is a huge place* [for the ethos of the PA communities] *but I don't think there is room being made, a place where that could be. Theoretically it is a very important place to happen, but it is not as if we have progressed from those ideas of that time. I don't think people have advanced that much in their ideas about the psyche. Laing was always trying to understand what madness was and how it came about. He was not trying just to treat it. So how have we progressed scientifically, so we now work with DNA and the reasons why someone is diagnosed schizophrenic, do we figure out what is wrong with our DNA*

so we can correct it? The genetic argument, Laing replied to many times, but the thing is, statistically it [the DNA hypothesis of mental illness] *does not hold water, but they keep bringing it up ... So we have not progressed in the sense of a linear line; going in one direction. I mean primitive societies, we have learned how they should progress, how to become more civilised, how to become like us, how to have television, telephones, machinery. Somehow this thought has replaced a lot of mythological thought which was part of ancient societies which was put together very beautifully. That has been replaced with a very shallow form of scientism ...*

Debbie

And of course, from the perspective of the topological study of borders, in relation not only to geographical boundaries, but also conceptual boundaries, a shallow scientism casts out potentially creative avenues and narratives which sustain and help human life flourish; creativity (and ability to go beyond fixed boundaries) in a dwelling space, amongst our fellow men and women and with ourselves, is a liberation from a fixed border or narrative. If the dominant narrative is, for example, 'fixing mental illness', the horizon or border only settles upon this space. If there is nothing other than this border, and the space within this border is a shallow scientism, then such a curtailing of creativity and exploration surely leads to a grotesque impoverishment? This is perhaps why, in other societies and cultures, broader, more fluid, colourful and creative forms of life and narratives lead to healthier and happier ways of life (Burckhardt, 1992; Guenon, 2007; Liedloff, 2004; Balibar, 1999; Hyde, 2007). The creation of a border, geographical or conceptual, creates and produces expectations. This can be thought of on one hand as helping to find one's way, but it also closes off the creation of making one's own way. This difference is subtle, but has far-reaching effects in the realm of mental distress; people lose their way precisely because the 'way' is already prescribed and cuts off any possibility of deviation, liberation and creativity. This is pertinent to the narrative of Debbie. Debbie had tried all the 'prescribed routes' (i.e., psychiatric care, medication, supported housing etc.) before coming to the PA house, which did not offer such a narrow scientistic prescribed route.

Debbie: *I did not have any expectations, I just hoped that I could live somewhere, you know, I was in a rut, things were not getting any better, so*

> *it was just hoping that things got better ... but not really knowing how ... or you know ... knowing there is just nowhere to go. I had tried everything ... I had no other options really ... you just stay miserable and ill, or try something else.*
>
> *... my main problem was (a psychiatric disorder) and I had been in hospital loads of times and all it really taught me was to stay out of hospital. All I learned was that there was no point in going through that again. I didn't learn anything so I learned to keep myself out of hospital, but I had not learned how to live life so to speak. I just learned how to survive and that's not enough really ... not enough for me anyway. Some people get to that point and they chug along, thinking it can be OK but I think I kind of stayed at that level for quite a few years, not really being well, but not ill enough to be in hospital and you know, nothing changes. Therapy was OK but even that was not enough and I think the only thing that would have been enough was living with other people.*

Her narrative above seems to elicit the idea that conventional prescriptive psychiatric treatment did not foster the opportunity for creativity to help her *imagine* herself on a level where there were other routes beyond the borders of the medico-scientific paradigm (which had been applied to her). However, although not prescriptive in its ethos, the house for Debbie, paradoxically, did present a border, metaphorically speaking, whereby the edges of and geography of this ethos, because they were unknown, fluid, and constantly in flux, did make Debbie feel trapped. She mentioned how people left the house as they could not stand such a non-prescriptive border and/or such a confrontation. The extract below from Debbie's interview describes this scenario, and highlights the paradoxical nature of the house experience.

> Debbie: *Probably for 90 per cent of the time absolutely awful* [her experience of the house]. *But then that's how it is – it's a horrible place because you can't run away from it. Basically I think most people find ways of running away from things in their life. In life you know, you can do that, you can avoid everything if you wanted but in the house unless you leave the house, but don't really want to do that because you have got nowhere really else to go. It's just like being trapped.*

BS: Really?

Debbie: *But in a positive way, in the long run, but it is a kind of trap. I mean you have to be bad enough ... I mean lots of people did leave because they came across things that they found very difficult* [to deal with] *and if you don't want to face them then you just leave and people did leave but maybe that's because they were not desperate enough to go through it. But I think it only works if you are very desperate and you have nowhere else to go ... you know ... that's your option ... to stay and deal with stuff. It's like unless you are at your lowest point it probably won't work, if you still think there are other options that might be easier, then you'll probably leave and that was quite interesting. I saw quite a lot of that. I knew people who thought if I went off and did this or went off there and did that it would be better ...*

BS: You said it was like hell?

Debbie: *Yeah, I don't remember it being like that. I saw it as a positive thing. In the last year or so I felt really good. Obviously it helped me in my life. I've got everything I ever wanted and that is purely down to the house, so I have happy thoughts and feelings about it, but most of the time I was living there I had thoughts about it being hell and wanting to leave. But when I was quite ready to leave I wanted to stay! You know when you're happy to stay that's when you're ready to leave.*

BS: Paradoxical?

Debbie: *Completely because you have got nothing to hide from anymore, you've got nothing to run away from anymore.*

Debbie also highlighted how creativity was fostered in such a non-prescribed PA house environment, despite being at one's lowest ebb.

Debbie: *Again, I think it's going to your lowest point and finding a way out of it, finding a new way out of it.*

The honesty of the perplexed and the honesty of perplexity

The idea that one has to be ready for such an experience, of finding one's way, despite it being paradoxically difficult was described by Debbie. She alludes to the desire of the existence of a protected bordering where difficulties would be spared from her.

> Debbie: *... you are in a vulnerable position and ideally you would like some nice warm cosy place to live and be protected and it* [the PA house] *was completely the opposite. You had more to deal with than most people. I came out of it fine, but I think some people found it pretty distressing and maybe some did not ... I can't talk for others ... I guess it has the potential to be quite damaging, people can be very aggressive.*

Again, later in the interview, Debbie alludes to the lack of borders which elicit a freedom. Interestingly, she refers to such freedom as being associated with a home. This idea ties into Cooper's (in Cooper et al., 1994) idea of autorhythmia and Heidegger's (1971) idea of dwelling, where the idea of what constitutes home and dwelling (in contrast to an institutional context) is the opportunity to flourish in one's own creativity in how one leads one's life without a prescription of how to live one's life, even if this can (and always will for everyone) create some kind of suffering, but a suffering which is unfortunately the human condition.

> Debbie: *Helpful things* [about living in the house] *were like, you could stay there as long as you liked, they did not throw you out, living with other people, having the house meetings, having the therapists always there. Really they were always brilliant whether you liked them or not at the time. They were always there. I guess the freedom ... you had a certain freedom ... You had a lot of freedom to do anything else you wanted really ... I mean you never get to stay (X) years in other places* [in reference to the length of time she stayed in the PA community house]. *I guess it was a home. It wasn't just a hostel or whatever. It was a home. It was never meant to be a short-stay place. It was meant to be somewhere where you made your home. That was very positive. They always encouraged you to feel at home, do what you want in your home.*
>
> *Unhelpful* [things about living in the house]: *I think was the amount of therapy, but again I don't know if that was unhelpful at all. I think it just felt unhelpful at the time but that might have just been*

> *because you wanted to do something else instead of doing therapy every day all the time. I can't really think of unhelpful things. I mean I know a lot of the time you want to leave and stuff, but I don't think that would have been helpful. I can't really think of any unhelpful things. Maybe things like leaving was very difficult, but I don't think it could have been made any easier.*

Debbie commented later on the inevitability of human suffering, which I believe is being banished by the mental health hygiene movement: e.g., cognitive behavioural therapy, and the government's Improving Access to Psychological Therapies programme for example. This highlights the danger of the constrictive nature (of banishing certain aspects of human experience) of medico-scientific borders and the subsequent psycho-pathologisation of human living, which, ultimately, creates a stifling non-human living environment. This is obviously congruent with Heidegger's (1977) prophecy about the dangers of technology applied to problems of human living; i.e., the danger of humans becoming objectified and losing their ability to assert their subjectivity.

> Debbie: *Well, I don't know, it's always easier to say in hindsight isn't it because I am happy I can't think of anything else I would rather have apart from what I have. So none of it has been easy. I don't think you ever leave and think your life is fine. I mean I definitely felt I have been helped without a doubt, but I mean years after leaving it was still difficult and I had difficult times. I think you learn when you are in the house when you are having difficult times they pass, things change and get better, even if you just sit still you sort of have this attitude that when things are really awful I would just sit still and just wait and time would pass, then I would go to bed and the next day I would be better or I don't know, things always changed. I just learned that in the house, if you did not run away it would still get better, even if you did nothing. I think the house therapists were into this thing you know* [the positivity of not running away from mental distress and staying with it]. *People often think they have to do something to change, however actually I think I learned how not to do anything and that things would change and that they would change by themselves. I don't know what I am on about (laughs).*

> ... *That is something very important that I learned in the house; just tolerate my own feelings of badness and not try to make them go away. And yeah, they pass on their own, and when that happens over and over again even when you have left the house you just think, oh well, I'll just have to wait for this to pass and when you feel better you can try again.*
>
> ... *I don't think there is an easy solution. It is not a miracle cure, you still have to do a lot of work even when you leave the house, that is how it happens, just by experiencing it, you learn from your experiences, and then you have those experiences and that's how you carry on.*

Towards the end of our interview Debbie summed up her wonderful philosophical outlook, touching upon many of the points I have discussed throughout this book.

> Debbie: *It's just the capacity to learn, if you have not got that ... if someone has helped you to learn that, to learn from life, to cope with the knocks and scrapes and things like that then you can carry on.*
>
> ... *You know, the humdrum, accepting the humdrumness of life, that's what it's about. For me, I have worked god knows how many years to get to this point, so for some people they would think that this is just ordinary life, this is not any achievement or anything, it just happens to them. Like my friends think, this is how everyone's life is. They don't think twice about it, but I am very conscious that it is an achievement and I think it probably makes me happier a lot of the time. Happier because I get moments where I think ... wow ... isn't this great! I am really lucky. Maybe other people don't think how lucky they are.*

Lyn

The issue of borders and boundaries in relation to the definition of the self was present in my interview with Lyn. It seems clear from how she described her experience that she found the demand, consistent with societal and cultural norms, for strict dichotomous self-definition (e.g., patient–therapist, depressed–non-depressed, sane–insane) difficult and perhaps unhelpful. The loosening of boundaries regarding the need for such self-definition seems to have given her a more authentic experience. This is unlike psychiatric establishments where dichotomous self-definitions such as patient–doctor or sane–insane are used and act as psychological boundaries and foreclose other possibilities of self-definition, or the loosening of strict self-definition.

> Lyn: *I had a really hard time trying to define myself as helper or a depressed person. I realised later and at the time as well that my life depended on being in the house. I look back on it and think I probably would have ended up in a psychiatric hospital like a lot of my friends did in those days … having the validation was incredibly important that whatever I was experiencing was real, having the camaraderie and for me the intellectual stimulation, the incredible rigour of it all.*
>
> *… There was no staff, everybody was all in it together, except whoever the house therapist was, who was paid to come around to the house. But anybody else there who had any illusions that they were an intern* [trainee therapist] *or anything else were shredded constantly. You know, it was a 'you are just one of us' kind of thing. And it* [this blurring of boundaries] *was true and that's what kept me there because of the authenticity of it all.*

Interestingly, the topic of borders and the pursuit of self-definition or the project of self-definition were subverted when Lyn realised that her own creative path involved moving away from the defining of the boundaries of her own self-definition, and instead not paying attention to her self-definition. Lyn's discovery of her path very much echoes Lacan's idea of moving away from a symbolic discourse where the imaginary is dominant, and Wittgenstein's idea that language (involving definitions of the self) is an entrapment (Lacan, 2007; Wittgenstein, 1980).

> Lyn: *I think there are some people for whom those diagnoses seem to fit a bit and within those people there are people who do very well in a structured environment and people who don't. What you find out is that even if you subscribe to some theory that there are some people who are psychotic and they are different from you and me, suppose you subscribe to that, they are not all that different and at the bottom of it it's all understandable* [people in mental distress]. *This is the gift I got from being in the PA house, being in it, being on the edge of my own madness, which in my case was depression.*

> *... So the other thing that I really learned from being in the PA house was that the path out of depression is service to others. I really got that and that served me over the years. Yeah, I was really depressed and suicidal but this woman over here or this woman over there* [in the house], *they were literally fighting with the devil for their life in that moment. And I said to myself, OK, I can come out of my depression for a moment and then help in a way that wasn't ego-based; it was being with them, and they were with me. It was quite amazing.*

This idea of moving away from a deceiving symbolic discourse or an overly close affinity with one's imaginary ego-ideal of self or self-definition was clearly expressed by Lyn under the topics of shamanism and initiation. This is fascinating, for clearly the traditions of shamanism and initiation as expressed in many cultures and societies (e.g., Sufi or monastic cultures; see Kalweit, 1987; Kingsley, 1999, 2003) do engender a path where egoistic borders of self are cast asunder as a way of becoming more whole, or as Plato or Parmenides (Plato, in Cooper, 1997; Geldard, 2007) might say, becoming aware of the indefinable oneness of existence or the ineffability of existence.

> Lyn: *... The shamanism that was flying around here* [in the PA House] *consciously and unconsciously ... Ronnie* [Laing] *was certainly a shaman. I mean the shaman walks between two worlds ... the daily experience of ego-shattering* [living in the house and having one's assumptions and one's being challenged] *is again shamanic. That is the truth about what shamans are* [what they do: shattering one's ego] *... once a year they* [shamans] *stand there and yank out their own hearts and let the vultures eat it so they can be reborn and that's what was going on in the PA house ... you had to walk between two worlds to survive ... and when you have had these experiences ... you've got it ... what they say about the shamans is that you have to go through things like that* [personal suffering and illness]. *I think that's what things like depression are; it is a shamanic initiation.*

Echoing Debbie's views, Lyn later described how the flux of the borders being present in the house and the unpredictability of daily life facilitated a creativity that was a very different experience to what one would encounter within a psychiatric milieu.

> Lyn: *It gave me a foundation so that when I did have a major depressive episode later, I didn't think that I had to go to hospital. I understood what it meant and I think that must be true … I think that the people that were there were loved, supported, had incredible insight, had conversion experiences, which they would never have had if they had been drugged up and in a psychiatric hospital … one thing I have is this visceral memory of the feeling of waking up* [when living in the PA house] *and thinking, what will be happening today? Because it was not predictable and I think that unpredictability was the authenticity and you would get up in the morning and come downstairs; there might be nobody there, it might be empty or there might already be people down there smoking cigarettes …*

Our conversation then came upon the topic of love and the heart in human flourishing in dealing with mental distress, from which one can suppose from this position, creativity and freedom to roam (and create and re-create our own borders) are present, and the flux of the borders between self and other is very much in attendance, which I believe may be a crucial ingredient in moving away from a failing symbolic discourse, opening oneself up to a place beyond discourse, in a Levinasian (see Levinas, 1998, 2007) hinterland, where the call from the *Other* always comes first before any violence from an imaginary agenda in the Lacanian sense (Lacan, 2007).

> Lyn: *… the love and compassion in the household was tremendous* [from residents and therapists].

> BS: When I was doing my training I told my supervisor at the time, James Low, he has studied Buddhism, so he is into that sort of stuff … and I said to him, this job as a therapist … it struck me the other day when I was sitting with a patient and it actually struck me also as a result of an experience I had with my wife. You know, you are sitting opposite a person, another human being, and you look at them and a sudden realisation came over me (which has happened with patients and in other contexts with people) and I thought, oh my God, the fragility of this other person, it's actually quite painful to see it. And … you know what I am getting at … to revert to a more ego-bound

way of functioning kind of protects you from this painful realisation [of the fragility of the Other].

Lyn: *Exactly, you're right, your whole heart ... people who work in psychiatric hospitals. that I think are objectifying, they are just scared and what they are afraid of is their own heartache, their own fragility. They really have those experiences you're describing. You said it beautifully.*

... So that fragility and when you keep your heart open it's painful. That's what shamans are talking about. They pull their heart out and let the vultures pick at it. That's how you stay alive. There is a Leon Redler [a current PA therapist] *story that I heard him tell. There is a Buddhist saying, when you have an open heart, you can see your spine. So in other words that's your strength as opposed to ego. The fact that an open heart makes you weak or vulnerable, it doesn't. I think that's what we got* [learned in the house] *as opposed to ordinary psychiatric or psychological experiences* [objectifying ideas about mental health]. *We learned that an open heart is what makes it possible. What else was I going to do but open my heart? Well I got stabbed a few times, metaphorically speaking, and then you learn over the years to open it up. It's easier than not doing so.*

Cara

Of course, as I have reiterated throughout this chapter, it seems one has to be of a constitution to be able to withstand the experience of the house. As Thomas made clear as did other interviewees, a PA house experience is not for everybody. For Cara, her experience of the house was mixed. It was not altogether an unhelpful experience, but she felt she needed more of an opportunity to confide in somebody, though she expressed that the house experience, however difficult, was preferable to a psychiatric hospital. Interestingly, 'confide' is etymologically related to the idea of confidence, and for one to open one's heart to another takes courage as one needs the confidence to do so But Cara did comment on how, for some of her fellow residents whom she felt were not in the correct environment, that a more structured environment would have been more apt for them. She also alluded to the necessity of 'working together' to help each other out, which can be a risky affair.

> Cara: *I think it was helpful being there and also helpful in getting my children back. It was a lovely setting. One to one, and have the group* [in addition] *would have helped. Someone to confide in would have been helpful.*
>
> *... My first experience of being a patient in a psychiatric hospital had been following an overdose of sleeping tablets about 14 years before living in the PA house. I had also had two brief stays following the birth of one of my children seven years after my first admission ... On each occasion I'd taken my own discharge* [from the hospital]; *I can't bear to think of what might have happened to me if I hadn't ... The lack of privacy, bullying, and mystification* [in the psychiatric hospital] *is enough to drive anyone mad let alone the medication and ECT* [electroconvulsive therapy] *or the threat of it.*
>
> *... Of course it was much, much better* [the house compared to psychiatric care] *even though it was difficult. But unfortunately there was not the support to prevent two of our former housemates, C, an artist, probably diagnosed with bipolar disorder and A, whom I believe had been labelled with schizophrenia, dying in their mid-40s of the effects of major tranquillisers.*

Indeed Cara found the distress and interactions with residents upsetting because of their lack of readiness. However, even within such difficult contexts, Cara found aspects of her own experience to reflect upon which, it seems, made her more compassionate and thoughtful.

> Cara: *I think that is what is needed, one needs support like that. Also, it is very important to have a high ratio of people who have worked through their problems already living in the houses to prevent us from destroying each other. I am ashamed of some of the hurtful things I said to people under the guise of being honest.*

The difficult experience also helped Cara become more aware of aspects of her life, the history of her experience, and guide her to realisations and to understand what might have been more helpful. Out of the confusion and chaos that Cara experienced of the PA house environment, some form of clearing was engendered; it was a painful process, but this perhaps highlights that one can only *get there* by *going there*, however painful or difficult that may be; but certainly it is not a process that can be preordained by others.

Cara: *... Looking back, I realise that what I really needed was family therapy for myself and my children to help us heal the wounds of a long separation from which we still haven't recovered.*

Rose

Rose's experience of psychiatric care echoes the other interviewees' comments in many ways. Rose describes how the boundary and borders erected in the psychiatric context were stifling, and indeed how such borders were mystifying and lacked meaning for her, by 'furthering' herself from herself by the regime that she was exposed to.

Rose: *In the hospital in (a town) I saw an alternative psychologist. I can't remember why or how. He thought I shouldn't be in the place that I was. It certainly was furthering me away from the person I felt that I should be. I felt I was being treated sadistically and this precipitated panic breakdown. So being in that hospital furthered me from myself, not being in touch with who I am and that furthered me from myself. I heard about a place called the PA and I ran away from that hospital because I thought if I stayed there I would have been there until I was an old lady. The things that were happening there were furthering me into panic; not being treated like a human being, other people around me were complete and utter vegetables and suffering from tardive dyskinesia from the effects of antipsychotic drugs.*

However, the experience of the house, because of the volatile nature of the interpersonal dynamics, did not seem for Rose the place for her to find a more authentic way of being. The complete lack of 'structure' seemed anarchic in this period (at least for her – other residents I spoke to did not share her view). In essence she felt the house did not take care of or alleviate the vulnerability she felt.

Rose: *So I went to a house that was already divided. It was like being in family having dreadful rows. It was a very traumatic place to be in,*

> *especially having gone there in complete trust thinking it would be a place of security; it was a very, very scary place to be and there was not enough security to be had outwardly from anyone in there. The only security net I had was that at least I had a nook of my own and that was something. But there were a lot of strong characters in there that were vehemently against anyone else being there. So I was vulnerable and it was very difficult to survive in a place like that. I was attacked by someone. But there was no one I was able to talk to and express what was going on. It was worse than staying in a ... it was worse than the worst of dysfunctional families and I was there for three-and-a-half years ... it was the most anarchistic place. Anybody could do anything to anybody and get away with anything. It was certainly a very frightening place to be. It didn't do my panic attacks, my nervous anxiety, any good whatsoever.*

However, despite Rose's complaints, she highlighted one reason why the PA house may not have been particularly suited for her. It seemed Rose was attracted to a more spiritual way of living that was perhaps missing in the house. This is interesting as in early PA houses (i.e., Kingsley Hall) Buddhist ideas were very prevalent and integrated in much of the daily life of the house (e.g., morning meditation). Although she points out that not having a religious or spiritual agenda was itself a positive thing in some ways, as nobody was preached to, she still felt there was a 'lack' which she felt needed to be filled. I got the impression that there were or are other more appropriate places or networks where *her needs* would have been met. This in itself is a correct point for Rose to make; the house did not provide what she wanted but as a result of this she discovered what she did want. That in itself is a positive movement.

> Rose: *It's interesting ... I heard a story at the PA – 'Behold I have set before you an open door and no man shall shut it'* [a quote from one of the PA advertising leaflets, originally from The New Testament, Book of Revelation, 3:8]. *I wish there had been more of a philosophy based on spiritual disciplines in the house. I wish there had been* [more of a spiritual dimension in the PA house] ... *you know you* [the author, before our interview began] *talked about Buddhism ... I wish there had been more Buddhism or Christian people who believed in spiritual matters, the love of God and shown that to one another. But people didn't*

want to know about spiritual matters either. I think it's a shame that it [the house] *didn't work out.*

BS: I see what you mean ... the PA espouses a kind of Christian/Buddhist ethics, but it didn't seem to be there in the community from your perspective[6].

Rose: *No, no ... but even in the churches it is missing in some that I have experienced. We each have got to find our own way, our own path in our lives so at least there wasn't anyone there that was going to be badgered into anything. But I think it went too far the other way really. It could have been a middle ground. But there wasn't ... there was none of the help that you can get today. But there was none whatsoever. Nuff said!*

Endnotes

1. One most notable idea is the value in *The Dark Night of the Soul* (2003) espoused by St John of the Cross. The potential value of a depression being a positive alchemical and/or transformative vehicle for change, growth, and empowerment is regarded as abandoning the institutional 'duty of care' within psycho-technician circles (i.e., NHS, HCPC, PSA, CBT practitioners). This important experiential aspect of the human condition is being forgotten about in our modern times However, such things can never be completely banished and made not to exist, but they may be proscribed and fester so that they surface in perhaps destructive ways (e.g., the London riots of 2011), where feelings of material poverty are perhaps not recognised as the futility of searching for happiness through material consumption, but instead a calling to the 'Dark Night' where such materialistic yearning would be put firmly into perspective.

2. It has been suggested that the 'true' philosophy of Parmenides has been distorted and forgotten in the West (by some, but not everyone by any means) over the last two thousand years, while its value was embraced into the Islamic east, Sufism and the philosophy of Ibn 'Arabi (Kingsley, 1999, 2003).

3. *Différance* is the systematic play of differences, of the traces of differences, of the spacing by means of which elements are related to each other. This spacing is the simultaneously active and passive production of the intervals without which the 'full' terms would not signify, would not function (the *a* of *Différance* indicates this indecision as concerns activity and passivity, that which cannot be governed by or distributed between the terms of this opposition). From Derrida, J. (1982). *Différance: Margins of Philosophy*. Chicago & London, University of Chicago Press, p. 17.

4. See the Health and Care Professions Council's standards of competence and conduct for psychologists (see www.hpc-uk.org).

5. The imaginary referred to here is in terms of Lacan's theory of the Imaginary. The Imaginary is the field of images, imagination, and deception. The main illusions of this order are synthesis, autonomy, duality, and similarity. Lacan thought that the relationship created within the mirror stage, between the Ego and the reflected image, indicates that the Ego and the Imaginary order themselves are places of radical alienation. In other words, alienation constitutes the Imaginary order. This relationship is also narcissistic (see Lacan, 2006).

6. Throughout the history of the PA, many members have been interested in spirituality (e.g., Buddhism, Christianity, Zen, and Sufism) and its connections with the psychotherapeutic endeavour. This has been reflected in an indirect (or perhaps direct) way with the ethos of how many therapists (past and present) within the PA view the practice of psychotherapy.

Part 4

Summing up a necessarily incomplete project

Chapter Twenty-One

Meno, Montaigne and *Docta Ignorantia*

R.D. Laing once said, 'Is it possible to be a human being anymore?[1] Is it possible to be a person? Do persons even exist?' On the surface these might seem like simple questions to answer. One can say that a human is a biological entity and has a complex anatomical system, and that humans do x, y, and z from a physiological, anthropological, or psychological standpoint. However, such answers fall flat in relation to mental distress; they miss the mark, blindly flailing in the chaos of ratiocination trying to find its final end, destination, or mountain top, where all will become clear. As Plato said in the *Theaetetus* (Plato, in Cooper, 1997), there is no end, or final clarification (in logical terms) in such human matters; all we can do is go about our daily life in the knowledge (of not knowing) that we can never put a full stop to the sentence that is human life. Some find this unacceptable, some crazy, some even terrifying. However, as Lacan (2006) argues, this not-knowing is a terror that has to be faced head on; otherwise we become mad as a result of some delusion of our own omnipotence.

The Philadelphia Association (PA) houses have survived, and are surviving under the constant brutal attack and questioning regarding the reasons for their existence and the reasoning behind their existence, to be held to account, to justify themselves, primarily in terms of their efficacy and productivity in relation to curing people and their financial viability. To my mind these can be, in certain contexts, important questions, but they are not the most important questions. From the interviews I conducted with ex-residents of the Philadelphia Association communities, I feel it is clear that the PA houses are a paradox, because they represent an approach that questions or puts into question the dogma of the medico-scientific regimes of certainty about mental distress. Such questioning involves: How can one love another? How can one be there for another? How can one be happy? How can one set another free? How can one be free? These questions, in our contemporary society and culture with its incessant cry for accountability, slip us by, become ignored, or are regarded as unimportant.

The PA houses uphold a different way of thinking – a discourse which allows the community residents to discover their own discourse or meanings beyond the dominant oppressive discourses circulating in our culture. This is why one must be wary of proffering theories of what one can expect about living in a PA community house, as *some* people might take such theories and use them thoughtlessly and apply them in a technological way to cure mental illness, missing the point that the PA houses try to allow an individual's subjectivity to flourish without the demands of ideological opposition and totalisation.

This concurs with the French analyst and psychiatrist Yves Cartuyvels (2006) who argues for the importance of the keeping open of *other* possible discourses which a 'psychoanalytic' way of working – and/or an existential-phenomenological and many other ways – *can* facilitate. Indeed, contrary to this way of working, the utopian CBT revolution, the government's IAPT programme, the new *DSM* (*DSM-5*, APA, 2013), the push for evidence-based practice in psychology and psychiatry, and NICE guidelines of mental health, sweeping our lands, demonstrate quite clearly that such state apparatuses are culturing out *free* thinking that does not, or cannot be, included in their all-subsuming oppressive, constrictive, and totalising discourse. This totalising discourse must be adhered to via various state mechanisms, and if one does not adhere to these mechanisms, punishments will be meted out; this is clearly ideological cleansing, however subtle it looks.

To give an example: when a patient disagrees with a psychiatrist about the neurochemical or cognitive basis of depression, the diagnosis of depression, and the neurochemical or cognitive psychotherapeutic treatment they are offered and receive, this is their right in trying to find meaning for themselves – and it is a valid questioning or questing; neurochemical and cognitive theories and treatments for depression are very much questionable (see Healy, 2003; Moncrieff, 2003; Wampold, 2001; Westen, Novotny & Thompson-Brenner, 2004). However, if such a patient refuses such a diagnosis and aborts whatever neurochemical or cognitive treatment regime in favour of another way, they are not out of the woods. The diagnosis and treatment of depression will be on their medical records and this may have some bearing on future possibilities for employment. Even if this person disagrees with the idea of the *DSM* diagnosis of depression (that they did not 'have' such a mental disorder as depression), a future employer will not take the word of the person that they did not 'have' depression. It will stay on that person's record like indelible ink; the medical gaze and its far-reaching influence is unavoidable. Surely it is within one's rights to disagree with the 'official' diagnosis of depression, considering the shaky evidence of the neurochemical and cognitive basis of depression, and have it removed from any records if one comes to the conclusion that it is incorrect?

Fortunately as I see it, the masters of mental health do not and cannot ever have a monopoly of what counts as *real meaning* of how it is to live and live through mental distress. If attempts are made to bring such a monopoly into being, as is surely happening in the United Kingdom today and in many parts of the Western world, these attempts amount to a political ploy for social control.

Certain discourses, for example, the *Diagnostic and Statistical Manual of Mental Disorders* (*DSM-5*) (APA, 2013), destroy other ways of conceptualising meaning. Considering Lacan's arguments regarding his discourses of the master and the university (Lacan, 2007), the symbolic of the *DSM* discourse is regarded as cast iron; words are taken as entities, these entities are taken as facts, and as a result of the proliferation of *DSM* diagnoses in the media, the *DSM* discourse becomes solidified into the symbolic/language of the public. However, such a covering-over and domination of the symbolic prevents one from contributing to the meaning-making of the world. What the *systematisers* cannot accept is that there may be many meanings or even that there is no final meaning; the symbolic continually evades the variety of the real (Lacan, 2007; Derrida, 2004). Why is the realisation of a questionable or imperfect symbolic such a terror? Is it such a terror? For many it is a terror; we live in a society where risk prevention is paramount, where avenues of alternative thought and searching for alternative meaning are outlawed, and where the questioning and traversing of ideological borders (e.g., patients questioning the psychological and psychiatric masters' ideas about the psychological and neurochemical basis of mental disorder) are forbidden and not taught in any of our state educational contexts.

As Cartuyvels (2006) eloquently describes, from a psychoanalytical position (or one could say an existential, phenomenological, or deconstructive position), a subject is immersed in language, which can be alienating in terms of freedom and one's own truth (see Wittgenstein, 1980). However, the subject condemned to the alienating aspects of language is consequently invited to question their language, the meaning of their life in relation to language, and the role of their own responsibility in relation to this predicament. The subject is marked by a lack and a desire, which does not lend itself to ever being completely educated, controlled, normalised. The truth or truthfulness of one's own meaning is out there (or right there already), but it is not predetermined by a manufactured and reified discourse like the evidence-based approach in psychology and psychiatry; one's individuality cannot ever be subsumed under such a totalising discourse as the evidence-based approach which is used widely in the UK's mental health establishments and government's projects.

The evidence-based approach (e.g., IAPT; *DSM-5*, APA, 2013) is a vision of humans as inherently social, oscillating between the regimes of self-management and self-control, subjugated by the mental hygiene regime of self-control, and dominated by the quest for wellbeing, efficacy and efficiency. Such a strategy may be profitable in terms of neoliberal capitalistic concerns – being a productive and social human being – but such a system defies alternate ways of being, and does not itself question its own system. Ultimately, such a strategy is alienating and imprisoning.

Cartuyvels (2006) warns us not to confuse pain (in the medical sense of getting rid of or reducing pain) and suffering when one thinks of mental distress. Of course it is understandable if one has a broken leg and one needs morphine to alleviate the pain, but when one is suffering from distress of a mental kind (although mental pain can be embodied in many ways) it could be too hasty to run to a cognitive behavioural therapist for some cognitive restructuring, or to a doctor for antidepressants, because both treatments can negate the meaning of the person's suffering. In other words, suffering may be legitimate as a way to discover meaning, but this takes time and patience, which is allowed if one stays in a PA house; I think that the interviews of ex-PA residents at the very least showed that this is allowed to take place.

Struggling to understand a new language is a form of suffering – it may drive one to despair – but if one halts the process of learning by prematurely aborting the suffering attached to learning, one will not learn or discover any further. One has to go through the suffering of finding meaning in the new language (and perhaps continue to suffer in a different way). This is a crude example, but I hope it highlights that we need to work at being reflexive and be critical of all the conditions the symbolic imposes upon us, be that from our family or from wider society, and this includes the symbolic discourse of mental health, of which from the Lacanian perspective (Lacan, 2007) seems to be that of the discourses of the master and the university ; where subjectivity is annulled as a result of obeying the discourse of the master of mental health or idealising an impossible truth system in the hope that it will be fruitful via the discourse of the university (e.g., depression is caused by low serotonin and/or negative cognitive structures). One has to think about the interviews with the ex-PA residents; suffering per se continued in those who got a lot out of their stay, while those who aborted it prematurely or did not get as much out their stay perhaps continued to suffer in a different way; struggle and suffering is the key it seems. The human condition necessitates suffering to a large degree to enable one to live 'fully'.

In response to a culturing out of suffering, or psycho-phobic aversion to mental distress, Cartuyvels (2006) describes some of the arguments that the adherents of the '*thérapies cognitivo-comportementales*'[2] put forward in the book *Le Livre Noir de la Psychoanalyses* (Meyer, Borch-Jacobsen, Cottraux, Pleux & Van Rillaer, 2006). These arguments rest upon dogmatic statements which range from the criticism that psychoanalysis cannot be tested empirically and psychoanalysis cannot be falsified (thus creating jobs for the boys), to accusations that Freud was a liar. However, Cartuyvels, rebutting these shallow claims, argues that psychoanalytic foundations of working are heuristically and incomparably richer than the terms of reference of, for example, scientific psychology, whose arguments are linked to staggeringly questionable statements of truth (i.e., depression is an illness) and inventing arbitrary cut-off points of what is depressive illness and what is not.[3] In other words, describing what is normal and what is abnormal. Cartuyvel's conviction is that human beings are specifically beings of meaning and language, and psychic suffering calls to this dimension.

This idea is pertinent to the project of the PA community houses and what they allow residents to encounter: their own meaning and their own language, and the meaning of others and others' language. In terms of the rich heritage of psychoanalytic, psychotherapeutic and philosophical thinking that places like the Philadelphia community houses are inspired by, it would be fair to say that the adherents of the '*thérapies cognitivo-comportementales*' have not recognised the depth of thinking that this heritage reaches back into. This is a way of thinking far beyond evidence-based practice of psychotherapy and psychiatry and is hundreds and even thousands of years older than scientific and academic psychology and psychiatry. One just needs to browse the literature of philosophers such as Parmenides, Plato, Montaigne, Heidegger, and Derrida, just for starters, and one begins to see how meaning and language have been the grist to the mill and how the project of psychoanalysis, psychotherapy, existentialism, and phenomenological thinking has its roots in something other than a neoliberal capitalistic project of defining what is normal, what is illness, and beyond the naïve idea of using techno-calculative methods to improve the human lot. Is this not for the good?

Plato's dialogue, *Meno*, which speaks directly to the experience of those who have lived in a PA house in many ways, is a wonderful example of an anti-technological stance to psychotherapy and an anti-system of psychotherapy. In *Meno*, Socrates and Meno debate the nature of virtue and whether it can be taught. Socrates concludes this dialogue:

> ... virtue would be neither an inborn quality nor taught, but comes to those who possess it as a gift from the Gods which is not accompanied by understanding, unless there is someone among our statesmen who can make another into a statesman. If there

> were one, he could be said to be among the living as Homer said Tiresias was among the dead, namely, that 'he alone retained his wits while others flitted about like shadows'. In the same manner such a man would, as far as virtue is concerned, here also be the only true reality compared, as it were, with shadows.
>
> (Plato, in Cooper, 1997, p. 897)

Like Lacan's hysteric (Lacan, 2007), a man searching for virtue from a teacher or somehow believing he has the inborn quality of it (perhaps by tapping into it through computerised CBT techniques) is flitting about in the shadows, believing there is a technical way to get what he wants; one would only be shadowboxing with illusions in such a case. The understanding of the 'Statesman' from Plato is the understanding of a technical endeavour of how to go about obtaining virtue; today the 'Statesman' is in a role of the CBT therapist, bio-psychiatrist, or logical-positivist therapist, having knowledge of the cure. (The 'Statesman', because he is the expert, should lead the polis, except that he really does not have this expertise: he only appears to know; see Cooper, 1997.) But as Plato shows in *Meno*, virtue comes to those as like a gift from the Gods and thus one's belief in having virtue is far different than being able to have knowledge of it. Therefore one has to find one's own *mind*, or perhaps be content in the idea that no imposed symbolic discourse can ever give one *the true answer*. In other words the art of conversation (and point of the dialogue) of Socrates in *Meno* is to teach the slave to give his own speech its own true meaning.[4] However, as Plato shows in *Meno*, one *cannot teach* someone to find their own meaning/discourse, just as one cannot teach someone good mental health, or force someone through various techniques to be cured from *mental illness* (which is a common occurrence today), because if one did this, the result is the creation of a 'slave'. Hopefully the reader can see, as expressed by the interviewees' comments, finding one's *own mind* was integral to the experience of living in a PA house; nothing was taught or prescribed out of a desire to bring about 'cure'. The PA and its houses open up a space where people can dwell and let their own subjectivity flourish, leading to their *own cure*.

On a similar note, Montaigne, from his essay 'The Art of Conversation', describes how conversation is a dialectic – an art (much like psychoanalysis and psychotherapy) where thoughtless reasoning and cogitation, slavishness to doctrine and dogma, and deferring to the wisdom of the other (or as Lacan (2006) would say, to the one supposed to know), leading to universal judgements, is a lax and dangerous path to take. Montaigne appeals to the *ordinary* in living a good life; an ordinariness that is beyond truisms of the academy dictated to the masses or a force-fed dogma of how we should live, and which leads us into absurdity. Montaigne describes:

> Take an arts don; converse with him. Why is he incapable of making us feel the excellence of his 'arts' and of throwing the women, and us ignoramuses, into ecstasies of admiration at the solidity of his arguments and the beauty of his ordained rhetoric! Why cannot he overmaster us and sway us at his will? Why does a man with his superior mastery of matter and style intermingle his sharp thrusts with insults, indiscriminate arguments and rage? Let him remove his academic hood, his gown and his Latin; let him stop battering our ears with raw chunks of pure Aristotle; why, you would take him for one of us – or worse. The involved linguistic convolutions with which they confound us remind me of conjuring tricks; their sleight-of-hand has compelling force over our senses but in no wise shakes our convictions. Apart from such jugglery they achieve nothing but what is base and ordinary. They may be more learned but they are no less absurd ... In my part of the country and during my own lifetime school learning has brought amendment of purse but rarely amendment of soul.
> (Montaigne, 1991, p. 1050)

Later on in the chapter 'On the Art of Conversation' Montaigne outlines why Socrates debates not for the sake of debating, but for the sake of the debater; to show the debater that ultimate truisms are ungraspable in how to go about living a good life. Montaigne, like Socrates (Cooper, 1997), Ibn 'Arabi (Chittick, 1989), Derrida (1997) and Lacan (2007), espouse the *Docta Ignorantia*; the doctrine of wise or learned ignorance as coined by the fifteenth-century philosopher and theologian Nicolaus Cusanus (2007). The idea of *Docta Ignorantia* is very important to psychotherapy and psychoanalysis; the position of an effective analyst or therapist is not to be the one who knows, but rather the one who can be formative for the subject; for the analyst to accept that he does not know anything about the analysand except for what the latter's own words, or signifiers, reveal. This position of wise ignorance is important to hold because, as Montaigne points out in his essay on experience, being dictated to in how to live one's life (i.e., to gain happiness or health) furthers one from oneself, or replaces one set or schemata of information to live slavishly by with another.

This state of affairs according to Montaigne is foolish and he describes why this is so in his lengthy essay, 'An Apology for Raymond Sebond' (Montaigne, 1991), an essay in honour of *Docta Ignorantia*. He describes how a person who abides by learned ignorance is somebody who is content to realise that all human knowledge is as nothing compared to that of infinity which is God; learned ignorance never claims to know, or aspire to know beyond what one can know. In essence, learned ignorance is a way or a path away from cogitation or reasoning to gain *health*: reasoning and cogitation towards unrealistic goals, that is, certainty. I am certainly not saying that reasoning and cogitation are bad per se; reasoning and cogitation performed to find out what we do not know is essential to reach or practise *Docta Ignorantia*. This position is unlike cognitive behavioural therapy or the government's IAPT utopian dogma, whose techniques focus on cogitation and reasoning about *things* (e.g., happiness) that cannot ever be truly *known*; reasoning about happiness cannot ever lead one to *know* happiness like one knows the length of a table top (Wittgenstein, 1980; Heaton, 2010). One can say 'I am happy' and explain why one is happy, but such reasoning ultimately fails to translate into a technical procedure where one can reproduce happiness. Ultimately happiness is not an object that can be manipulated via calculative or technological thought (Heidegger, 1977).

I feel that the narratives from the ex-residents of the Philadelphia Association communities showed a form of learned or wise ignorance; residents are led to the houses in mystery and perplexity. This perplexity is not suffocated by the house therapists by a schema or doctrine of knowledge to lead people out of their perplexity. Instead it seems they are led to arrive at a position to be able to know what is possible and what is not possible; this is not psycho-scientific knowledge, but a path back to, or the creation of, an increasingly forgotten art of living. This art of living is a very different prospect than that proffered by the mental hygiene movement which intends, it seems, through its psycho-techniques, to maintain the status quo of how one sees the world or keeps it within pre-ordained boundaries, usually through the eyes of the *master* (i.e., bio-psychiatrist or logical-positivist psychologist).

To some, these ideas may not seem convincing or relevant to how one should think about dealing with mental distress. However, we must go further to tease out why *Docta Ignorantia* is relevant, by showing why a materialistic way of dealing with and conceptualising mental distress is actually anti-democratic and contra freedom, despite on the surface of the CBT, IAPT and NICE wasteland, it might look promising. From this I hope to show how an anti-materialistic stance towards dealing with mental distress is actually towards freedom, respectful of the subjectivity of a person, and what the Philadelphia Association communities engender, or at least leave open for people to take up.

For a starting point, to outline a critique of the materialistic stance towards mental distress, one can do no better than look to Jean-Paul Sartre. Sartre (1972) argued that materialism (especially in its psycho-scientific guise) had the effect of understanding (and consequently of treating) people like objects. In other words materialism thinks of people as an assemblage of quantitative qualities and phenomena, just as one would think of the qualities of a stone, chair, or table. Sartre wanted to get away from this type of thinking and reconstitute a way of thinking that regarded a person as an ensemble of values distinct from a materialistic way of regarding people. Such an argument against materialistic thinking may seem self-evident, but this slips people by when they fall hook, line and sinker for the medico-psycho-scientific agenda of the CBT, IAPT, and NICE dogmatic utopias and how these institutions facilitate and disseminate the idea that a person is a mechanical or technical object to be manipulated, destroying and imprisoning our subjectivity.

As Clotilde Leguil-Badal (2006) describes, one of the major paradoxes of our times concerns the status of the subject. A result of the progress of science and how it currently stands today is that a new definition of the subject and subjectivity has been imposed; this is a subject that is composed of a material, organic substrate, or a cognitive machine which is observable, i.e., the brain's neurochemicals or the results of cognitions expressed in a psychometric questionnaire. Leguil-Badal describes from a political standpoint how subjectivity is being wiped out, paradoxically because we supposedly live in an age where freedom, democracy, and the rights of the individual are held up as values. On the one hand we have 'freedom' and the 'human rights to freedom and to be what we want when we want', yet on the other hand we have the neurosciences, the computer-like/information processing discourse of CBT and the IAPT discourse (cognitive reprogramming for the unemployed), and the psycho-scientific ideology of mental health and illness from the likes of NICE. These discourses of power banish subjectivity, as neuroscience and the science of mental health rule and guide subjectivity. This creates a landscape with no landmarks; science is the big authority on how we feel, think, and experience; subjectivity is written out of the picture. If people become unhappy they blame it on their neurons or cognitions. In turn they demand happiness, assuming it is a human right and that such a thing as an imaginary ideal of mental healthiness is possible; this is a big double-bind, a vicious circle. The human spirit is never seen in an MRI scan or in the results of a cognitive psychology laboratory experiment measuring reaction time to depressive or negative stimuli (e.g., negative words paired with self-referent words). What is missed in this discourse is that the subject exists by their speech, their silence, and their actions, not by a scientific knowledge or discourse. The subject *existing* in the here and now is being forgotten about; we are increasingly defining ourselves by an abstract fictitious scientific *Weltanschauung* in order to become free, but by defining ourselves by science we paradoxically give up our liberty and subjectivity.

The rise of brain science and cognitive science is in many ways actively denouncing the creativity of the subject. The subject (or psyche) is being absorbed into theories about the working of the brain and cognitive theories of inner schematic representations, with the result that activities such as psychoanalysis and psychotherapy which adopt the approach of *Docta Ignorantia* are being made out to be redundant and useless. Cognitivism and the neurosciences have taken away the unity of the individual or rather the possibility to know oneself as an impossible unity; in other words to know that we cannot *know* everything about how to live a human life (i.e., that the *Self* is an illusory construction, or one can at least put the idea of the *Self* into question). In other words, the cognitive-neuroscientific discourse invites one to conceive of oneself as a machine, as a processor of information, receiver/perceiver of stimuli, and a network of neuronal interactions. As a result, the *Self* becomes a concrete, material, and ideological entity.

The government's cognitive neuroscientific agenda is spreading like an empire. As is the case with empires, borders are blurred; one does not know where one culture starts and another begins. Aspects of subjective experience are being cultured out under the homogeny of the empire. The 'treats' of the empire, unlimited freedom, democracy, health, and happiness, come with a price tag – one's subjectivity and the wherewithal to cogitate and reason the ability to recognise the limits of what we can know and what we cannot know. We become as Deleuze and Guattari (2004, pp. 165–184) put it, a 'cancerous body without organs' (i.e., our embodiment of a stultifying, crippling, fixed discourse). Yes, we are a brain; we do have neurochemicals, and we think, but we are primarily subjects, subjects able to question the very idea of our subjectivity, our knowing and unknowing. In continuing to hold to this, a hold onto suffering, which, however difficult it may be to accept, is as much a part of what it is to be a subject (or foundation-*less* subject) as it is to live, be happy and to die. 'The Borromean knot' (Lacan, 2006, pp. 671–702) that is being tied by the cognitive-neuroscientific empire results in such suffering or free subjectivity not being allowed to flourish.

The people I interviewed, guided by their struggles, their subjectivity, unhindered by ideological borders (or protected from hindering ideology to some extent by the asylum of the houses), are allowed the increasingly outlawed freedom to be confronted by their distress and to try to make sense of their world and life. This is a gift of asylum and it is a privilege to be able to do this in this day and age. There are far too many people ready to shore up, correct, cure any distress. Like Montaigne (1991) described in his essay on experience, one has to find one's own balance through trial and error. Indeed, we have to be allowed to err. Our subjectivity is not some kind of machine that needs fixing like a broken computer. It is much more complex than that.

The Philadelphia Association houses are an incomplete project. There can be no technical theory presented for the implementation of what the PA houses try to offer. What can be described, and I hope to have shown this, is only the ordinary, free confrontation with perplexity, suffering, joy, tears and all the other things that are part of ordinary life. Yes, the projects of the houses themselves are informed by philosophical and psychoanalytic theories, but they are influenced by the school I believe that R.D. Laing belonged to: the school of learned ignorance.

A school of learned ignorance cannot have a curriculum, a theory, or an agenda, or tell others how to do it; one can only let a person speak or not, if that is what a person chooses. Therein lies its secret, its liberating function, which is none other than the word spoken (or not spoken) by its residents and its therapists: the freedom to *testify* truthfulness. Life is a paradox, as Kierkegaard (1975) expressed; on the one hand we have reason and cogitation, and on the other hand, reason and cogitation fall to pieces. Montaigne (1991) described this as nature's way – we cannot reason our way out of our human state, we cannot explain the reason we exist, we just have to accept this and go along with what is our human fate and ordinariness. But, it seems today, nobody can face being ordinary. Many people seem to aspire to cosmetic psychological or cosmetic psychopharmacological methods to bypass our *thrown-ness* into the world. Such people have fallen into a dangerous trap where such yearning can never yield the '*objet petit a*' as Lacan (2007) might say.

I do not feel this is necessarily a morbid idea – to live by *Docta Ignorantia* – it can be a path of liberation. One cannot explain to someone who cannot get *it*, how to get *it*. When Freud (2001) was asked by a patient how long it would take for the cure to take place he replied by inviting the patient to walk (metaphorically speaking). It was only then that Freud would be able get a sense of how the patient would progress on the way to what one could call living a good life. We can only invite people to walk, and let them walk freely. If we protest and tell them they have to walk down a certain road in a certain way and that we are the master of this road, they will never learn to walk by themselves. The people who I interviewed were invited to walk; some found their feet, some better than others. I will leave you with a poem from Rilke which sums up much of what I have endeavoured to capture and what the ex-residents of the Philadelphia Association houses conveyed to me: the importance of struggle, ordinariness, patience, the gift of being able to testify freely, and *Docta Ignorantia*.

> You darkness, that I come from,
> I love you more than all the fires
> That fence in the world
> For the fire makes
> A circle of light for everyone,
> And then no one outside learns of you.
>
> But the darkness pulls in everything:
> Shapes and fires, animals and myself,
> How easily it gathers them! –
> Powers and people –
>
> And it is possible a great energy is moving near me.
>
> I have faith in nights.
>
> (Rilke, 'You Darkness', 1981, p. 21)

Endnotes

1. Quote taken from the album by The Winchester Club, *Negative Liberty*, from the track 'R.D. Laing (Little Chemical Straightjackets)'.
2. Cognitive behavioural therapy.
3. It must be noted that psychoanalytic theory and thinking can also be criticised for being dogmatic and mystifying and can share some of the criticisms that cognitive behavioural theory attracts. See John Heaton's (2010) book *The Talking Cure: Wittgenstein's therapeutic method for psychotherapy* for an excellent critique of psychoanalytic theory.
4. One could say the modern slave is under the spell of the discourse of the master or the university as described by Lacan. See Lacan's *Seminar XVIII*, 2007.

Coda

Over and above a conclusion, a final word necessitates what: truth, wisdom, or closure? This is not my goal and has not been my goal in writing this book. Hadot (2002) describes how the goal of the ancient Greeks was not to discern a final truth, or the production of ultimate knowledge, but to be a practice in helping to form the individual; a praxis which is unending, a praxis that has no definite curriculum, nor can be taught in the modern academic sense. It was also a practice to help judge and criticise effectively. Therefore, the Greeks were not against discursive reasoning, as was the author of *De Docta Ignorantia*, Nicolaus Cusanus; discursive reasoning is essential to get us to the place where we can discern what we can know and what we cannot know. I am in accord with such an idea. Therefore, I hope the reader will not confuse what I have written about with the notion that thinking, cogitation, or reasoning is useless. To become enamoured by such an idea would set oneself up as being accused of advocating 'anything goes' or lazy thinking, especially within the psychotherapeutic context. I hope the reader will digest or re-read the testimony of ex-residents of the Philadelphia Association communities: but do not judge their testimony too harshly, or put a full stop to end any unfinished business you think needs a closure, or pose any unnecessary questions. But, to end, a point for meditation, drawing on Marcuse (2002, p. 36) quoting Perroux (Francois Perroux, *La Coexistence Pacifique*, 1958, p. 600):

> The slaves of developed industrial civilization are sublimated slaves, but they are slaves, for slavery is determined 'neither by obedience nor by hardness of labour but by the status of being a mere instrument and the reduction of man to a thing'.

And some appropriate last words from Nicolaus Cusanus himself:

> ... but since the natural desire in us for knowledge is not without a purpose, its immediate object is our own ignorance. Nothing could

be more beneficial for even the most zealous searcher for knowledge than his being in fact most learned in that very ignorance which is peculiarly his own; and the better a man will have known his own ignorance, the greater his learning will be. It is in bearing this in mind that I have undertaken the task of writing a few words on learned ignorance.
(Nicolaus Cusanus, *On Learned Ignorance*, 2007, p. 8)

Appendix

Pro-forma questions for PA houses research

Return completed questions to: Bruce Scott
Address:
Telephone:

PA research questions pro-forma

Please write on a separate piece(s) of paper.
Please write as much as you can with as much detail as possible.
Only disclose information that you feel comfortable with.
All information given is confidential – your identity will not be disclosed on any research paper/report.

1. How did you hear about the (PA) houses?
2. What was your motivation for going to live in a house?
3. What was the procedure for getting into the house?
4. What did you know about the PA houses?
5. What was your experience of living in the house? (e.g., meetings, therapy, therapists, day-to-day life, practicalities of living in the house, ethos.)
6. How long did you stay? (e.g., Was any length of time stipulated? Was it too long, too short, just right etc?).
7. Did you have experience of other communities and other mental health services? How did the PA houses compare to these other places?
8. What did you find helpful about living in the house?
9. What did you find unhelpful?
10. What was difficult about living in the house?

11. Is there anything you wished you had got out of living in the house but did not receive?
12. Any thoughts, reflections, recommendations that you have since leaving the house?
13. Would you recommend the experience of living in the house for people suffering from mental distress? Why?
14. Is it any better/worse (the PA houses) than the alternatives? If so why?
15. And anything I have left out?

Thank you for your time.

References

Almond, I. (2004). *Sufism and Deconstruction: A comparative study of Derrida and Ibn 'Arabi.* Abingdon: Routledge.

American Psychiatric Association (APA). (2013). *Diagnostic and Statistical Manual of Mental Disorders: Fifth edition.* Washington, DC: American Psychiatric Association.

Anonymous. (2001). *The Cloud of Unknowing* (Trans., A.C. Spearing). London: Penguin Classics.

Balibar, E. (1999). *At the Borders of Europe.* Lecture delivered October 4, 1999 at Aristotle University, Greece. Retrieved from http://makeworlds.net/node/80

Baudrillard, G. (1994). *Simulacra and Simulation.* Ann Arbor, MI: University of Michigan Press.

Beck, A.T. (1967). *Depression: Clinical, experimental, and theoretical aspects.* New York: Hoeber.

Beck, A.T. (1976). *Cognitive Therapy and the Emotional Disorders.* New York: International Universities Press.

Beck, A.T., Steer, R.A., & Brown, G.K. (1996). *BDI-II: Beck Depression Inventory manual* (2nd ed.). San Antonio, TX: The Psychological Corporation.

Buber, M. (1970). *I and Thou* (Trans., W. Kaufmann). New York: Touchstone.

Burckhardt, T. (1992). *Fez: City of Islam.* Cambridge: The Islamic Texts Society.

Cartuyvels, Y. (2006). Le livre noir de la psychoanalyse. In J.-A. Miller (Ed.), *L'anti Livre Noir de la Psychoanalyse* (pp. 216–223). Paris: Éditions du Seuil.

Chittick, W.C. (1989). *The Sufi Path of Knowledge: Ibn al-'Arabi's metaphysics of imagination.* Albany, NY: State University of New York.

Cooper, D.G. (1978). *The Language of Madness.* London: Allen Lane.

Cooper, J.M. (Ed.). (1997). *Plato: The complete works.* Indianapolis, IN: Hackett Publishing Company Inc.

Cooper, R., Friedman, J., Gans, S., Heaton, J.M., Oakley, C., Oakley, H., & Zeal, P. (1994). *Thresholds between Philosophy and Psychoanalysis*. London: Free Association.

Cusanus, N. (2007). *On Learned Ignorance* (Trans., G. Heron). Eugene, OR: Wipf and Stock Publishers.

Deleuze, G. & Guattari, F. (2004). *Anti-Oedipus: Capitalism and schizophrenia*. London: Continuum.

Derrida, J. (1982). *Différance: Margins of philosophy*. Chicago & London: University of Chicago Press.

Derrida, J. (1995). The secrets of European responsibility. In *The Gift of Death* (Trans., D. Willis). Chicago: University of Chicago Press.

Derrida, J. (1997). *Deconstruction in a Nutshell: A conversation with Jacques Derrida* (edited and commentary by J.D. Caputo). New York: Fordham University Press.

Derrida, J. (2004). *Positions*. London: Continuum.

Derrida, J. (2007). *Psyche: Inventions of the other: Volume 1*. Stanford, CT: Stanford University Press.

Dunne, J. (1993). *Back to the Rough Ground: Practical judgment and the lure of technique*. Notre Dame, IN: University of Notre Dame.

Evans, C.B. (1924). *Meister Eckhart: Works*. London: J.M. Watkins.

Feyerabend, P.K. (1975). *Against Method*. New York: Verso Books.

Foucault, M. (2001). *Madness and Civilization*. Abingdon: Routledge.

Foucault, M. (2007). *The Order of Things*. Abingdon: Routledge.

Foucault, M. (2008). *Psychiatric Power: Lectures at the Collège de France, 1973–1974*. New York: Palgrave Macmillan.

Freud, S. (2001). *Volume XII: Case History of Schreber, Papers on Technique and Other Works*. In *The Standard Edition of the Complete Psychological Works of Sigmund Freud*. London: Vintage UK Random House.

Geldard, R.G. (2007). *Parmenides and the Way of Truth*. New York: Monkfish Publishing Company.

Gittings, R. (1966). *Selected Poems and Letters of Keats*. London: Heinemann Educational Books.

Goffman, I. (1974). *Asylums*. London: Pelican.

Gordon, P. (2010). *An Uneasy Dwelling: The story of the Philadelphia Association community houses*. Ross-on-Wye: PCCS Books.

Guenon, R. (2007). *The Crisis of the Modern World*. Varanasi, India: Indica Books.

Hadot, P. (2002). *What is Ancient Philosophy?* (Trans., M. Chase). Cambridge, MA: The Belknap Press of Harvard University.

Hadot, P. (2006). *The Veil of Isis: An essay on the history of the idea of nature* (Trans., M. Chase). Cambridge, MA: The Belknap Press of Harvard University.

Healy, D. (2003). Lines of evidence on the risks of suicide with selective serotonin reuptake inhibitors. *Psychotherapy and Psychosomatics, 72,* 71–79.

Heaton, J.M. (1998). The enigma of health. *European Journal of Psychotherapy, Counselling, and Health, 1*(1).

Heaton, J.M. (2010). *The Talking Cure: Wittgenstein's therapeutic method for psychotherapy*. Basingstoke: Palgrave Macmillan

Heidegger, M. (1962). *Being and Time* (Trans., J. Macquarrie & E. Robinson). Oxford: Blackwell.

Heidegger, M. (1971). *Poetry, Language, Thought* (Trans., A. Hofstadter). New York: Harper & Row.

Heidegger, M. (1977). *Basic Writings*. San Francisco: Harper.

Heidegger, M. (1998). *Parmenides* (Trans., A. Schuwer & R. Rojcewicz). Bloomington, IN: Indiana University Press.

Heidegger, M. (2001). *Zollikon Seminars: Protocols – conversations – letters* (Ed., M. Boss; Trans., F. Mayer & R. Askay). Evanston, IL: Northwestern University Press.

Hyde, L. (2007). *The Gift: How the creative spirit transforms the world*. Edinburgh: Canongate Books.

Itten, T. (1977). Standing and Understanding Living in a Therapeutic Community. Unpublished dissertation, Bachelor of Arts in Social Science, Middlesex University.

Kalweit, H. (1987). *Shamans, Healers and Medicine Men*. London: Shambhala.

Kierkegaard, S. (1975). *Philosophical Fragments* (Eds. and Trans., H.V. & E.H. Hong). Princeton, NJ: Princeton University Press.

Kingsley, P. (1999). *In the Dark Places of Wisdom*. Inverness, CA: The Golden Sufi Centre.

Kingsley, P. (2002). *Reality*. Inverness, CA: The Golden Sufi Centre.

Lacan, J. (1999). *The Seminar of Jacques Lacan, Book XX: On Feminine Sexuality, the Limits of Love and Knowledge, 1972–1973* (Trans., B. Fink). New York: W.W. Norton and Co.

Lacan, J. (2006). *Écrits*. New York: W.W. Norton & Co.

Lacan, J. (2007). *The Other Side of Psychoanalysis. The Seminar of Jacques Lacan: Book XVIII* (Trans., R. Grigg). New York: W.W. Norton & Co.

Laing, R.D. (1967). *The Politics of Experience and the Bird of Paradise*. Harmondsworth: Penguin Books.

Laing, R.D. (1972). *Asylum*. A film by Peter Robinson. Kino Video.

Laing, R.D. (1977). Philadelphia Association information leaflet.

Layard, R. (2006). *Happiness: Lessons from a new science*. London: Penguin.

Leguil-Badal, C. (2006). Être ou ne plus être & Sur le cognitivisme. In J.A. Miller (Ed.), *L'anti-Livre Noir de la Psychoanalyse*. Paris: Éditions du Seuil.

Levinas, E. (1998). *Otherwise than Being* (Trans., A. Lingis). Pittsburgh, PA: Duquesne University Press.

Levinas, E. (2007). *Totality and Infinity* (Trans., A. Lingis). Pittsburgh, PA: Duquesne University Press.

Liedloff, J. (2004). *The Continuum Concept: In search of happiness lost*. London: Penguin Books.

Macmurray, J. (1939). *The Boundaries of Science: A study in the philosophy of psychology*. London: Faber & Faber.

Marcuse, H. (2002). *One-Dimensional Man*. London: Routledge.

Meier, C.A. (2003). *Healing Dream and Ritual: Ancient incubation and modern psychotherapy*. Einsiedeln, Switzerland: Daimon Verlag.

Meyer, C., Borch-Jacobsen, M., Cottraux, J., Pleux, D. & Van Rillaer, J. (2006). *Le Livre Noir de la Psychoanalyses*. Paris: Les Arènes.

Moncrieff, J. (2003). A comparison of antidepressant trials using active and inert placebos. *International Journal of Medicine, 12,* 117–127.

Monk, R. (1990). *Ludwig Wittgenstein: The duty of genius*. London: Vintage.

Montaigne, M. de (1991). *The Complete Essays* (Ed. & Trans., M.A. Screech). London: Penguin Books.

Mullan, B. (1995). *Mad to Be Normal: Conversations with R.D. Laing*. London: Free Association Books.

Nietzsche, F. (1974). *The Gay Science* (Trans., W. Kaufmann). Toronto: Random House.

Perroux, F. (1958). *La Coexistence Pacifique: Vol. 3*. Paris: Presses Universitaires.

Purcell, M. (1998). *Mystery and Method: The other in Rahner and Levinas*. New York: Fordham University Press.

Rapoport, R.N. (2001). *Community as Doctor: New perspectives on a therapeutic community*. Abingdon: Routledge.

Redler, L. (2000). R.D. Laing's contribution to the 'treatment' of schizophrenia: Responsible responses to suffering and malaise. *The Psychoanalytic Review, 87*(4), 561–589.

Rilke, R.M. (1981). *Selected Poems of Rainer Maria Rilke* (Trans., R. Bly). Toronto: Fitzhenry & Whiteside.

Rumi, J. (1994). *Signs of the Unseen: The discourses of Jalaluddin Rumi* (Trans., W.M. Thackston, Jnr). Boston: Shambhala.

St John of the Cross. (2003). *Dark Night of the Soul.* New York: Dover Publications.

Sartre, J.-P. (1972). Dear Comrades! Preface from the book: *SPK: Turn illness into a weapon.* Heidelberg: KRRIM.

Speck, R. (1974). *The New Families.* London: Tavistock Publications.

Stein, C. (1995). *The Parmenides Project.* Retrieved from: http://harveybialy.org/files/The_Parmenides_Project.pdf

Wampold, B.E. (2001). *The Great Psychotherapy Debate.* New York: Lawrence Erlbaum.

Westen, D., Novotny, C.M. & Thompson-Brenner, H. (2004). The empirical status of empirically supported psychotherapies. *APA Psychological Bulletin, 130*(4), 631–663.

Wittgenstein, L. (1961). *Tractatus Logico-Philosophicus* (Trans., G.E.M. Anscombe & B.F. McGuiness). London: Routledge and Kegan Paul.

Wittgenstein, L. (1980). *Remarks on the Philosophy of Psychology: Volume 2* (Trans., C.G. Luckhardt & M.A.E. Aue). Oxford: Blackwell.

Index

A
alienation, state of 7–8
Almond, I. 171, 174, 179, 181, 184
American Psychiatric Association (APA) 15, 24, 28, 218, 219, 220
antidepressants 220
anti-method 44, 165
    search for 22*ff*
    statement for 41–3
Aristotle 4, 36, 45, 172
asylum 5, 8–11, 12, 13, 17, 78, 80, 226
Asylum (film) 111, 119
autorhythmia 8–11, 112, 113, 114, 165, 190, 191, 192, 203

B
Balibar, E. 12, 200
Barnes, Mary 111, 117, 119, 135, 190
Baudrillard, G. 164
Beck, A.T. 24
'Being' x, 4, 29–35, 43, 44, 47, 163
'being with' 9, 34, 137, 152, 158
Berke, Joseph 119
Borch-Jacobsen, M. 221
Boss, M. 10, 11
Buber, M. 6, 22
Burckhardt, T. 200

C
capitalistic
    culture 26
    neoliberal 220, 221
Cara (interviewee) 63*ff*, 209–11
'care in the community' 5, 14, 15, 17–18, 97
Carr Gomm community care 18

Cartuyvels, Y. 218, 219, 220, 221
Chittick, W.C. 174, 176, 181, 223
cognition 36, 39, 43
cognitive behavioural therapy (CBT) 5, 23, 33, 38, 45, 46, 184, 204, 224
cognitivism 38, 226
communities
    of the Philadelphia Association (see Philadelphia Association)
    other therapeutic 11, 12, 14, 15, 20, 118, 131, 173
control, staff 14–15
'controlled observation' 27
Cooper, D.G. 8, 13, 27
Cooper, J.M. 4, 40, 165, 170, 171, 207, 217, 222, 223
Cooper, R. 7, 9, 16, 203
Cusanus, N. x, 163, 165, 171, 223, 229, 230

D
Dark Night of the Soul 46, 133, 137, 213
data collection 48
David (interviewee) 120*ff*, 193–6
Debbie (interviewee) 139*ff*, 200–5
deconstruction 190, 196
    Derrida's notion of 178, 189
Deleuze, G. 15, 182, 198, 226
Derrida, J. x, 12, 19, 38, 163, 165, 171, 174, 175, 176, 178, 179, 181, 184, 189, 191, 192, 193, 198, 214, 219, 223
diachrony 32, 33, 34, 43, 45, 164
diagnosis 12, 24, 106, 152, 218
Diagnostic and Statistical Manual of Mental Disorders (*DSM*) viii, 15, 17, 18, 24, 28, 72, 177, 218, 219, 220

Index

Diana (interviewee) 53ff, 175–9
Différance 189, 214
discourse (Lacanian)
    of the analyst 169, 171, 172
    of the capitalist viii
    of the hysteric 7, 16, 40, 169, 170, 171, 222
    of the master 7, 16, 18, 40, 169, 170, 171, 178, 220, 228
    of the slave 18
    of the university 7, 16, 18, 40, 169, 170, 171, 220, 228
Docta Ignorantia viii, x, *passim*
    introduction to 163–4
Dunne, J. 4, 36, 172

E

Eckhart, M. 4
Evans, C.B. 4
evidence-based approach 218, 219, 220, 221
existential/ism 218, 219, 221

F

Feyerabend, P. 16, 19, 24, 42, 43, 163, 164
Foucault, M. 12, 13, 14, 15, 41, 42, 46
Freud, S. 227
Friedman, J. 9

G

Geldard, R.G. 47, 165, 181, 199, 207
Gittings, R. 173
Goffman, I. 15
Gordon, P. 14, 164, 234
grief 13
Guattari, F. 15, 182, 198, 226
Guenon, R. 200

H

Hadot, P. 164, 229
Health and Care Professions Council (HCPC) 5, 16, 17, 28, 45, 159, 180, 191, 213, 214
health, problem of 35–41
Healy, D. 17, 218
Heaton, J.M. 35, 36, 37, 38, 39, 46, 172, 184, 224, 228
Heidegger, M. 4, 5, 8, 9, 17, 28, 29, 30–2, 40, 44, 45, 164, 174, 181, 183, 199, 203, 204, 224

Hillman, James 134, 137
Huxley, Francis 153, 159
Hyde, L. 200

I

Ibn 'Arabi 171, 174, 176, 179, 181, 184, 213, 223
ignorance, learned (see *Docta Ignorantia*)
Improved Access to Psychological Therapies (IAPT) 5, 37, 180, 184, 218, 220, 224, 225
incomplete project, the 4–5, 227
interviewees, characteristics of 50
interviews
    analysis of 164–73, 174ff
    method 48–9
Itten, T. 8, 10, 11, 12, 14, 15

J

Joe (interviewee) 77ff, 180–1
Jones, Maxwell 15, 118
Julia (interviewee) 95ff, 183–4

K

Kalweit, H. 26, 207
Keats, J. 173
khôra 19, 32
Kierkegaard, S. x, 16, 17, 20, 21, 163, 165, 167, 169, 171, 227
Kingsley Hall 5, 8, 48, 50, 119, 196, 212
Kingsley, P. 26, 29, 46, 181, 199, 207, 213

L

Lacan, J. x, 7, 16, 29, 40, 46, 163, 164, 166, 167, 168, 170, 172, 178, 184, 198, 206, 208, 217, 219, 220, 222, 223, 226, 227, 228
Lacanian
    discourses (see discourse)
    framework 16
    theory of the Imaginary 214
Laing, R.D. 5, 6, 7, 9, 10, 21, 27, 119, 190, 217, 227, 228
language ix, 20, 31, 34, 46, 168, 206, 219, 221
Layard, R. 23, 24
Levinas, E. vii, ix, 5, 6, 29, 32, 33–4, 40, 41, 42, 43, 44, 45, 172, 175, 208
Liedloff, J. 200
logos 33, 34, 41, 42, 43, 45

239

Lyn (interviewee) 150*ff*, 205–9

M
Macmurray, J. 44
   philosophical psychology of 23–8
Marcuse, H. 229
master–slave dialectic 45, 46, 196
Meier, C.A. 26, 46
Meno 170, 221, 222
Merton, Thomas 133, 137
method/ology 22*ff* (see also anti-method)
   scientific 21, 22–3, 27, 31, 34, 42, 46, 137, 165
Meyer, C. 221
Moncrieff, J. 17, 218
Monk, R. 39
Montaigne, M. 123, 163, 165, 171, 222, 223, 226, 227
Mosher, Loren 131
Mullan, B. 5, 27, 127, 190

N
National Institute for Health and Care Excellence (NICE) 5, 17, 18, 28, 45, 218, 224, 225
negative capability 166, 171, 172, 173
neurochemical/s 7, 225, 226
   treatment 7, 218
neuroscience 219, 225, 226
Nietzsche, F. 5, 6
nigredo 135, 137, 198

O
Oakley, C. 16
ontology 29, 30, 32, 33, 41, 155 (see also 'Being')
Other (Levinasian) 28, 29–35, 44, 45, 47, 208

P
paradox, a necessary 19–21, 173
Parmenides x, 28, 29–30, 42, 43, 45, 47, 163, 165, 181, 183, 199, 213
Perroux, F. 229
Peter (interviewee) 127*ff*, 196–200
phenomenology 106, 118, 119, 153, 218, 219, 221
Philadelphia Association *passim*
   attitude to employment 14
   communities 11–16 *passim*
   ethos 8, 34, 48, 63, 85, 94, 101, 106, 111, 129, 130, 133, 143, 190, 198
   honouring of true asylum 11–16
   houses (list) 50
   philosophical underpinnings 5–7
philosophy, Western viii, 4, 24, 28–9, 33, 41, 43
phronesis 37, 39, 40, 41, 46
Plato x, 4, 19, 20, 29, 32, 34, 163, 165, 171, 207, 217, 221–2
   Dialogues 45, 170, 221, 222
Professional Standards Authority (PSA) 5, 16, 28, 213
progress, myth of 23–8
psychiatric truth 17
psychiatry (see also diagnosis, *DSM*, evidence-based approach)
   backlash against 27
   experience of 106, 178, 187, 195, 205, 210, 211
   and objectification 5, 6, 7, 8, 9, 157, 204, 209
psychoanalysis 171
   framework 88, 89, 221, 228
   praxis 172, 218, 219, 221
psychologism, problem of 29–35
psychology 23–8, 37, 137, 218, 221
psychopharmacology 25, 31
psychotherapy 5, 8, 9, 20, 21, 31, 221, 223, 226 (see also CBT)
Purcell, M. 32

Q
questionnaire, research 231–2

R
Rapoport, R.N. 15
Redler, L. 8, 111, 135, 157, 190, 209
'religion of comfortableness' (Nietzsche) 6, 7
research viii, ix, 12
   practicalities of this 48*ff*
   schema, a 163*ff*
   scientistic 22–45
Rethink (organisation) 12, 17
Richmond Fellowship 8, 12, 14
Rilke, R.M. 227, 228
Rob (interviewee) 84*ff*, 181–2
Roland (interviewee) 68*ff*, 176–80
Rose (interviewee) 91*ff*, 211–13

Rumi, J. 46

S
St John of the Cross 46, 133, 137, 213
Sally (interviewee) 103*ff*, 136–90
Sartre, J.-P. 17, 50, 224, 225
schema, research 163*ff*
scientific method, problem of 21, 22–3, 43
self-love 20, 21
service users 5, 15, 16
Simon (interviewee) 98*ff*, 184–5
Speck, R. 11
spiritual/ity 4, 63, 64, 94, 137, 212, 214
Stein, C. 29, 30
suffering ix, 5, 6, 10, 32, 41, 89, 165, 196, 204, 220, 226
Sufi/sm 44, 46, 135, 174, 207 213
Summerhill School 136, 138
synchrony 33, 34, 43, 45, 164

T
testimony vii, x, 229
Thomas (interviewee) 111*ff*, 190–3
treatment
    for mental distress 20, 37
    no 7, 8, 10, 164
    in psychiatric system 5, 24, 27, 36, 40, 45, 218, 220
    -punishments 12
    technicalisation of 7–8

W
Wampold, B.E. 218
Westen, D. 218
Western thought, origins of 28–9
wise unknowing (see *Docta Ignorantia*)
Wittgenstein, L. viii, 22, 36, 38, 39, 46, 163, 206, 219, 224, 228
wounded healer 134, 135

Z
Zen Buddhism 3, 21, 36

R.D. Laing: 50 years since The Divided Self
Edited by Theodor Itten and Courtenay Young
ISBN 978 1 906254 54 4

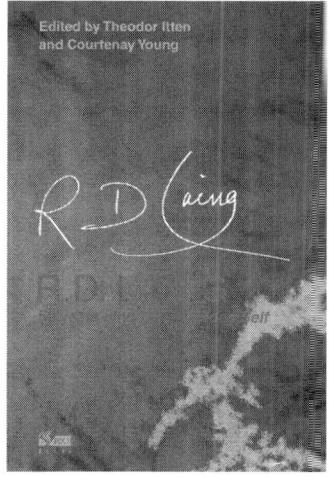

Collected in these pages are writings critically appraising Laing's life, work, frailties, brilliance, and his wide and varied influences over the last half century. You will find transcripts, memoirs, newly commissioned articles and a few previously published papers. Contributions have come from colleagues, friends and clients, as well as people who never knew him personally, yet deeply appreciate his work. Each is different in tone and character. Each captures something unique about Laing and his work.

An Uneasy Dwelling:
The story of the Philadelphia Association community houses
by Paul Gordon

ISBN 978 1 906254 24 7

Hundreds of men and women, whether formally designated 'mentally ill', or experiencing serious emotional distress to the point where they can no longer cope, have found in the Philadelphia Association's community houses a haven, a place where, in the company of others, they are allowed to go through whatever they have to go through in their own time and in their own way, free from the well-meaning interventions of psychiatry or family.

Despite the longevity and the radically different nature of the project, surprisingly little has been written about the work. This book is an attempt to correct that. It is in part a history of the houses as well as an account of how the houses work today and an exploration of their underpinning ethos.

Critical Examinations –
new series edited by Craig Newnes

Critical evaluation is an essential element of academic study. Any theory is only as strong as its capacity to withstand sustained critical examination of the assumptions it makes about the world. The individual volumes in this series, written by prominent experts and insider critics in their field, critically examine the theories and practices of the main branches of psychology in an accessible style.

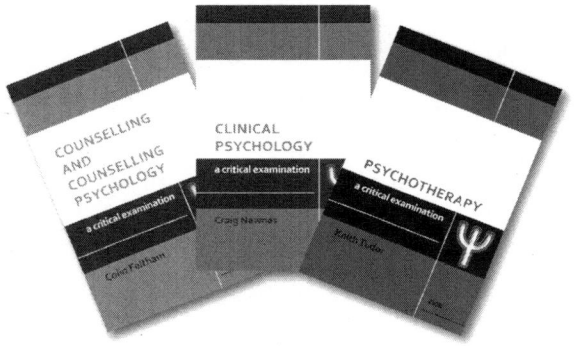

Counselling and Counselling Psychology: A critical examination
Colin Feltham
ISBN 978 1 906254 58 2
April 2013

Clinical Psychology: A critical examination
Craig Newnes
ISBN 978 1 906254 59 9
January 2014

Psychotherapy: A critical examinaton
Keith Tudor
ISBN 978 1 906254 61 2
(Spring 2015)